# Coaching Psychology Manual

## SECOND EDITION

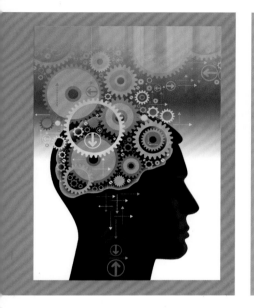

# Coaching Psychology Manual

**SECOND EDITION**

Margaret Moore

Erika Jackson

Bob Tschannen-Moran

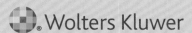

Wolters Kluwer

Philadelphia • Baltimore • New York • London
Buenos Aires • Hong Kong • Sydney • Tokyo

*Acquisitions Editor:* Michael Nobel
*Product Development Editor:* Staci Wolfson
*Editorial Assistant:* Tish Rogers
*Marketing Manager:* Shauna Kelley
*Production Project Manager*: David Orzechowski
*Design Coordinator:* Stephen Druding
*Artist/Illustrator:* Graphic World, Inc.
*Manufacturing Coordinato*r: Margie Orzech
*Prepress Vendor*: Absolute Service, Inc.

Second Edition

9 8 7 6 5 4

Printed in China

**Library of Congress Cataloging-in-Publication Data**

Moore, Margaret, MBA, author.
  Coaching psychology manual / Margaret Moore, Erika Jackson, Bob
Tschannen-Moran ; with the Wellcoaches Faculty team. -- Second edition.
    p. ; cm.
  Includes bibliographical references and index.
  ISBN 978-1-4511-9526-2
  I. Jackson, Erika, author. II. Tschannen-Moran, Bob, author. III.
Wellcoaches Corporation. IV. Title.
  [DNLM: 1.  Counseling. 2.  Health Behavior. 3.  Health Promotion. 4.
Motivation.  WM 55]
  R727.415
  610.73'7--dc23
                              2015018769

LWW.com

*This manual is dedicated to my wonderful husband, Paul Clark, a biotechnology patent attorney, who dreamed up the idea for me to start Wellcoaches in 1999 while I was a biotechnology executive.*

*Paul is the reason that my life and the lives of many thousands of coaches and their clients are now works of art.*

**Margaret Moore/Coach Meg**

# About the Authors

**Margaret Moore** (aka Coach Meg), MBA, is a 17-year veteran of the biotechnology industry in the United States, United Kingdom, Canada, and France. She served in executive roles at three companies which later joined Sanofi and served as CEO and COO of two biotech companies.

In 2000, Margaret shifted from high-tech medicine to build the field of coaching in healthcare and wellness and founded Wellcoaches Corporation—strategic partner of the American College of Sports Medicine, now a standard-bearer for professional coaches in healthcare and wellness. The Wellcoaches School of Coaching has trained more than 10,000 health and wellness coaches in 45 countries.

Margaret is co-founder (with Carol Kauffman) and co-director of the Institute of Coaching at McLean Hospital, Harvard Medical School affiliate and co-course director of the annual Coaching in Leadership and Healthcare conference offered by Harvard Medical School. Margaret's collaboration with Edward Phillips, MD, to create a Harvard Medical School CME program to teach physicians basic coaching skills led to the launch of the Institute of Lifestyle Medicine, now based at Joslin Diabetes Center, of which Margaret is an advisor.

She is a co-founder and co-leader of the National Consortium for Credentialing Health and Wellness Coaches which is delivering national standards and certification of health and wellness coaches to help catalyze the transformation of our healthcare system.

Margaret is a faculty member of the Harvard University Extension School, leading and teaching a coaching psychology program.

Margaret was born on a dairy farm northeast of Toronto where she attended a two-room school and learned to drive a tractor. She is a board member of the Boston Philharmonic Orchestra. Margaret lives in Wellesley, Massachusetts, with her husband,

Paul Clark, a prominent biotechnology patent attorney who patented the first genetically engineered animal, the Harvard mouse. She is both a U.S. and Canadian citizen.

*CME Course*

Harvard Medical School online CME course: *Prescribing Lifestyle Medicine for Weight Management* (basic coaching skills for physicians)

*Books & Book Chapters*

- *Organize Your Mind, Organize Your Life*, a Harvard Health book published by Harlequin (2012)
- Chapter 22: "Health and Wellness Coaching"; *The Complete Handbook of Coaching*, 2nd edition
- Chapter 27: "Health and Wellness Coaching Skills for Lasting Change"; *Lifestyle Medicine* (medical textbook), 2nd edition, 2013
- "Health & Wellness Coaching for Sustainable Change," Wegener/Fritze/Loebbert, Coaching-Praxisfelder

**Erika Jackson**, MLHR, MCC, BCC, is the VP of Operations and Training for Wellcoaches Corporation where she has gratefully served coaches for over 10 years in a variety of teaching and mentoring roles. Now leading the faculty and operations teams for the world's best coach training organization, Erika most enjoys the opportunity to improve processes that enable coaches to become more masterful, more quickly.

For the last 20 years, Erika has served a Human Resources and Organizational Development leader in the public and private sectors, ranging from a Fortune 500 organization to a local nonprofit. Erika has expertise in adult learning methodology and an expansive toolbox of teaching methodologies. She has consistently engaged in ongoing skill development through various coaching schools as well as concentrated study in appreciative inquiry and nonviolent communication. Erika is also qualified in the use of the Myers Briggs Type Indicator and is an instructor for the Harvard University Extension School, teaching coaching psychology courses.

In addition to her work with Wellcoaches, she is also the lead instructional designer and senior facilitator with ImprovEdge, designing "play with a purpose" leadership development experiences led by Ivy League graduates and professional actors based on the principles of improvisational theater.

Erika loves the arts and in her spare time runs a community theater, writes music with her husband, Theo, and performs in musicals. Most of all, she loves singing with her three children—Lo, Wren, and Elek.

**Bob Tschannen-Moran**, IAC-MCC (IAC), BCC, is the CEO and co-founder of the Center for School Transformation, president of LifeTrek Coaching International, and past president of the International Association of Coaching (IAC).

Bob is the co-author of *Evocative Coaching: Transforming Schools One Conversation at a Time* (2010, Jossey-Bass) and the ACSM/Lippincott Williams & Wilkins *Coaching Psychology Manual* (2010) as well as more than 700 articles and newsletters published in both print and electronic formats. Together with his wife, Megan, he co-authored the lead article in the October 2011 issue of *Educational Leadership* magazine, "The Coach and the Evaluator." Bob is an IAC Master Certified Coach, a CCE Board Certified Coach, a graduate of several coach training programs, and holds a Master of Divinity degree from Yale University.

Bob is active in Kiwanis and running. His family includes his wife, Megan, a professor of educational leadership at the College of William and Mary and a collaborator in LifeTrek Coaching International; his daughter, Bryn Rodriguez, a medical doctor in Las Vegas, and her husband Andres; as well as his son and daughter-in-law, Evan and Michelle Tschannen, who graduated from the University of Virginia with master's degrees in Systems Engineering and Special Education, respectively. These days, Bob finds the most delight in spending time with his three grandchildren: Everest and twins, Aliana and Amaya.

# Contributors

**Lori Gray Boothroyd, PhD, LP, PCC**

Faculty, Wellcoaches Corporation
Traverse City, Michigan

**Juli Compton, PhD, BCC**

Faculty, Wellcoaches Corporation
Boise, Idaho

**Gabe Highstein, PhD, RN**

Faculty, Wellcoaches Corporation
Faculty Emeritus, Wellcoaches Corporation
East Falmouth, Massachusetts

**Greg Hottinger, MPH, RD**

Faculty, Wellcoaches Corporation
Boulder, Colorado

**Erika Jackson, MA, MCC**

Vice President, Operations and Training,
  Wellcoaches Corporation
Carroll, Ohio

**Carol Kauffman, PhD, ABPP, PCC**

Assistant Clinical Professor, Harvard Medical
  School
Executive Director, Co-Founder, Institute of
  Coaching
Arlington, Massachusetts

**Kate Larsen, Executive Masters, MCC, BCC**

Faculty, Wellcoaches Corporation
Eden Prairie, Minnesota

**Christina Lombardo, MA, MCC, BCC**

Faculty, Wellcoaches Corporation
Powell, Ohio

**Sam Magill, MBA, MCC**

Faculty, Wellcoaches Corporation
Edmonds, Washington

**Kelly Davis Martin, MA**

Faculty, Wellcoaches Corporation
Sisters, Oregon

**Barrett McBride, PhD, MCC, BCC**

Faculty, Wellcoaches Corporation
Sacramento, California

**Margaret Moore, MBA**

Founder and CEO, Wellcoaches Corporation
Wellesley, Massachusetts

**Michael Pantalon, PhD**

Faculty, Wellcoaches Corporation
Hamden, Connecticut

**Robert Rhode, PhD**

Assistant Professor, Clinical Family and
  Community Medicine
Department of Psychiatry
University of Arizona
Tucson, Arizona

**Beverly J. Richstone, PhD**

Monument, Colorado

**Pam Schmid, BS, BCC, ACSM HFI**

Certified Executive Wellness Coach
Faculty, Wellcoaches Corporation
Clayton, North Carolina

**Michael Scholtz, MA**

Faculty, Wellcoaches Corporation
Hendersonville, North Carolina

**Gloria Silverio, MS, PCC, BCC**

Faculty, Wellcoaches Corporation
Delray, Florida

**Walter R. Thompson, PhD, FACSM, FAACVPR**

Department of Kinesiology and Health
Georgia State University
Atlanta, Georgia

**Darlene Trandel, PhD, RN/FNP, MSN, CPP, PCC**

Faculty, Wellcoaches Corporation
Chevy Chase, Maryland

**Bob Tschannen-Moran, MDiv, IAC-MCC**

Wellcoaches Faculty
Williamsburg, Virginia

**Jessica Wolfson, BS, PCC, BCC**

Faculty, Wellcoaches Corporation
Oakland, California

# Reviewers

**Terry Dibble**

Oakland University
Rochester, Michigan

**Matt Ferguson**

WebMD Health Services
Portland, Oregon

**Jennifer Guthrie, MS, CHES**

Independent

**Charlie Hoolihan, BA, CSCS*D**

Personal Training Director
Pelican Athletic Club
Mandeville, Louisiana

**Jeff Lynn, PhD**

Associate Professor
Exercise and Rehabilitative Sciences
Slippery Rock University
Slippery Rock, Pennsylvania

**Maureen McGuire, PhD, RN**

Associate Professor
Loretto Heights School of Nursing
Regis University
Denver, Colorado

**Darian Parker, PhD, NSCA-CPT**

Regional Account Director/General Manager
Club Ridges Fitness Center
Las Vegas, Nevada

**Jennifer Pintar, PhD, MPH**

Chairperson/Professor
Human Performance and Exercise Science
Youngstown State University
Youngstown, Ohio

**Leia Spoor**

Director of Health & Wellness
Baylor Health System
Dallas, Texas

**Tom Spring**

Director
Health Engagement and Community Relations
Health Alliance Plan of Michigan
Detroit, Michigan

**Troy Thomas, PhD**

Chief Academic Officer
U Train U LLC
Dallas, Texas

**Darlene Trandel, PhD, MSN, FNP/RN, CCP, PCC**

Family Nurse Practitioner, Clinical Specialist
ICF-PCC Certified Executive Health Coach,
    Consultant and Trainer
The Health and Well Being Institute, LLC
Chevy Chase, Maryland

**Eric Vlahov, PhD**

Professor
Health Sciences and Human Performance
The University of Tampa
Tampa, Florida

**Charles M. Ware, DHEd, MS, CHES**

Associate Faculty
College of Humanities and Science
University of Phoenix
Las Vegas, Nevada

**Rachelle Winkler**

Oakland University
Rochester, Michigan

**Heike Yates, ACE Certified Trainer**

CEO/Owner
HEYlifetraining Pilates & Wellness
Silver Spring, Maryland

# Preface

Wellcoaches Corporation, the American College of Sports Medicine (ACSM), and our growing community of coaches are building the foundation for the new professions of wellness coach, health coach, and fitness coach. Since Wellcoaches was founded in 2000, we have worked hard to establish the gold standard in coaching competencies in the healthcare, fitness, and wellness industries. Our integrity; commitment to the highest standards; and our passion, vision, and dedication are what bonds the Wellcoaches community together.

Having trained more than 10,000 coaches and now more than 1,200 coaches per year (all who have learned from previous versions of this manual), we've built the largest community of coaches in healthcare worldwide and the foundation to support a global industry that we hope grows to 100,000 coaches or more.

Although this manual, widely used by coach training programs and universities around the world, is now in its second edition, it represents only the beginning. The field of coaching psychology continues to rapidly evolve with our help. The way our coaching psychology curriculum has grown indeed mimics the way coaching works with clients. A clear vision has led to clear goals and impressive outcomes that continually stretch us in new and surprising ways. Since the publication of the first edition, our curriculum has matured into a robust and evidence-based protocol now published in nine research studies with many more to come.

We are teaching evidence-based coaching psychology to pioneering credentialed professionals in health, fitness, and mental health, enabling them to energize and empower clients to master health well-being. Together, we hope to make a dent in some of the toughest challenges of our times: the epidemics of obesity, sedentary lifestyles, stress, poor nutrition, and ever-rising healthcare costs.

## Organization

This manual comprises 12 chapters designed to provide the emerging coach with the knowledge needed to practice the skills necessary to perform the tasks required of a competent coach. The knowledge and skills outlined in this manual represent over 12 years of experience in educating and training 10,000 health and allied health and wellness professionals on how to coach. Each chapter provides sample coaching conversations to extend the translation of theory into practice.

The manual's coaching processes have been validated through dozens of coaching interventions and protocols. The manual supports the coaching science to practice content assembled by the Institute of Coaching at McLean Hospital, a Harvard Medical School affiliate, co-founded and co-led by Wellcoaches founder Margaret Moore. The manual also supports the national standards and certification set forth by the National Consortium for the Credentialing of Health and Wellness Coaches, co-founded and co-led by Wellcoaches founder Margaret Moore.

The first three chapters focus on becoming and being a coach. In Chapter 1, we explore definitions of coaching; describe coaching specialties; introduce scope of practice, ethical, and liability guidelines; and make the case for professional coaches trained in best practices. Chapter 2 discusses the key skills that generate the coaching relationship. Chapter 3 discusses coaching presence and introduces being skills and the importance of self-care.

The next two chapters examine ways to respectfully honor clients and "accept and meet them where they are." In Chapter 4 we introduce the constructs of compassion and nonviolent communication and their importance for coach self-care as well as supporting clients to better understand their emotions, needs, and drives. Chapter 5 provides tools rooted in positive psychology and appreciative inquiry for building of strengths and positive emotions as resources to support sustainable change.

Next, we provide a structural foundation for moving clients toward a vision for wellness or well-being, grounded in heartfelt purpose and meaning. Beginning with an examination of the importance and types of motivation, Chapter 6 describes the philosophies and tools of motivational interviewing for building self-efficacy. Chapter 7 explores the richness of the transtheoretical model and its cognitive and behavioral processes of behavior change.

Finally, we describe the tools and processes for facilitating the process of change. Chapter 8 discusses approaches to client assessment, followed by Chapter 9, which describes detailed approaches and guidelines for helping clients build visions and goals based on the creative and collaborative principles of design thinking. In Chapter 10, we then describe the heart of a coaching session, the generative moment, which represents the most powerful, creative, and engaging moments in coaching. Conducting coaching sessions, described in Chapter 11, provides step-by-step checklists that allow new coaches to get a head start in navigating coaching sessions.

And, in the spirit of lifelong learning, we close Chapter 12 with the introduction of a new model human thriving building on nine human primary needs, drives, values, and capacities.

The publication of this manual continues to help us realize our vision, which is nothing less than helping people take charge and master health and well-being on a large scale. To get there, large numbers of professionals will need to learn and master the principles and practices of coaching psychology presented in this manual. The more dedicated we are to "walking the wellness walk" and to assisting others on the journey through dynamic, growth-promoting coaching relationships, the more probable that our dream will become a reality.

## Features

Thank you for making the leap and working to become a world class coach who will make a big impact on the lives of many. We are delighted that you have joined the movement. We ask you to help us continue to define and meet the highest possible standards.

Margaret Moore (Coach Meg)
Erika Jackson
Bob Tschannen-Moran

# Acknowledgments

This manual represents the culmination of 15 years of work by many colleagues and collaborators. The first iteration of our manual was developed from 2000 to 2002 by Margaret Moore in collaboration with Steven Jonas, MD; Gabe Highstein, PhD; Juli Compton; Sheryl Marks Brown; Kate Larsen; Joan Price; and Tony Rodriguez. Important contributions from others followed quickly and include Walter Thompson, PhD; Robert Rhode, PhD; Lori Gray Boothroyd, PhD; Pam Schmid; and Jessica Wolfson. Gloria Silverio led a complete editing of the manual in 2006 as well as bringing in significant and new content.

Nearly a decade ago, Bob Tschannen-Moran and Erika Jackson spearheaded an enormous effort to expand the curriculum by integrating tenets of positive psychology, strengths-based change strategies, nonviolent communication, and relational flow (the intuitive dance of coaching). They also led the effort to structure the curriculum in accord with adult learning theory and to align the curriculum with our certification process, creating wonderful checklists and guides that are incorporated into the first edition of the manual in 2010.

We would not have completed the manual without the tireless efforts of the Wellcoaches operations team to support all of us including Blaine Wilson, Marilyn Thom, Julie Cummings, Angela Miller Barton, Sheryl Richard, Nicole Hansen, Ray Diveley, Robin Wilson, Kristin Lindstrom, and Kelly Noffsinger.

Most important, our coach trainees have contributed continually to the evolution and presentation of coaching skills and processes. They have challenged us to make them elegantly simple to practice and use.

All of us enjoy using these principles and practices every day to support both our own and our clients' health and well-being. Not only have we all undergone personal transformations, we are incredibly fortunate to be the partners in the small and large transformations that our clients experience. It's rewarding beyond compare. Coaching is our future.

Margaret Moore
Erika Jackson
Bob Tschannen-Moran

# Contents

**CHAPTER 1**    **Introduction**    **1**

*Part 1: Defining the Role of a Coach* . . . . . . . . . . . . . . . . . . . . . . . . . . . . . . . . . . . . 1
What Is Coaching? . . . . . . . . . . . . . . . . . . . . . . . . . . . . . . . . . . . . . . . . . . . . . . . . . . . . 1
Why We Need Health and Wellness Coaching . . . . . . . . . . . . . . . . . . . . . . . . . . . 2
What Coaching Is Not: The Expert Approach . . . . . . . . . . . . . . . . . . . . . . . . . . . . 5
Health and Wellness Coaching Research . . . . . . . . . . . . . . . . . . . . . . . . . . . . . . . . 7
How Coaching Works . . . . . . . . . . . . . . . . . . . . . . . . . . . . . . . . . . . . . . . . . . . . . . . . 7
APPENDIX A: What Brings Clients to Coaching? . . . . . . . . . . . . . . . . . . . . . . . . 10
*Part 2: Coaching Psychology* . . . . . . . . . . . . . . . . . . . . . . . . . . . . . . . . . . . . . . . . . . 11
What Is Coaching Psychology? . . . . . . . . . . . . . . . . . . . . . . . . . . . . . . . . . . . . . . . 11
Self-Determination: The End Game of Coaching . . . . . . . . . . . . . . . . . . . . . . . . 11
Four Coaching Mechanisms of Action . . . . . . . . . . . . . . . . . . . . . . . . . . . . . . . . . 12
*Part 3: Training, Scope of Practice, and Professional Guidelines* . . . . . . . . . . . . . 17
Becoming a Coach . . . . . . . . . . . . . . . . . . . . . . . . . . . . . . . . . . . . . . . . . . . . . . . . . . 17
Distinguishing Coaching and Therapy . . . . . . . . . . . . . . . . . . . . . . . . . . . . . . . . 20
Distinguishing Coaching from Other Professionals . . . . . . . . . . . . . . . . . . . . . 20
Liability and Scope of Practice . . . . . . . . . . . . . . . . . . . . . . . . . . . . . . . . . . . . . . . 21
APPENDIX B: The ICF Standards of Ethical Conduct . . . . . . . . . . . . . . . . . . . . 22

**CHAPTER 2**    **Coaching Relationship Skills**    **27**

Relationship: The Heart of Coaching and Growth . . . . . . . . . . . . . . . . . . . . . . . 27
Establishing Trust and Rapport . . . . . . . . . . . . . . . . . . . . . . . . . . . . . . . . . . . . . . . 29
Mindfulness . . . . . . . . . . . . . . . . . . . . . . . . . . . . . . . . . . . . . . . . . . . . . . . . . . . . . . . 32
Three Core Coaching Skills . . . . . . . . . . . . . . . . . . . . . . . . . . . . . . . . . . . . . . . . . . 34
Additional Relationship-Building Tools . . . . . . . . . . . . . . . . . . . . . . . . . . . . . . . 38

**CHAPTER 3**    **Coaching Presence**    **43**

Defining Coaching Presence . . . . . . . . . . . . . . . . . . . . . . . . . . . . . . . . . . . . . . . . . 43
Being Skills . . . . . . . . . . . . . . . . . . . . . . . . . . . . . . . . . . . . . . . . . . . . . . . . . . . . . . . . 44
Conveying Coaching Presence . . . . . . . . . . . . . . . . . . . . . . . . . . . . . . . . . . . . . . . 49
Coaching Presence as a Symphony of Strengths . . . . . . . . . . . . . . . . . . . . . . . . 49
Being Skills Tied to Strengths . . . . . . . . . . . . . . . . . . . . . . . . . . . . . . . . . . . . . . . . 53

**CHAPTER 4**    **Expressing Compassion**    **55**

How Coaches Handle a Client's Negative Emotions . . . . . . . . . . . . . . . . . . . . . 55
Exploring Self-Esteem . . . . . . . . . . . . . . . . . . . . . . . . . . . . . . . . . . . . . . . . . . . . . . 56
Self-Compassion: How to Suffer Well and Calm One's Inner Critic . . . . . . . . 57
Nonviolent Communication: A Model for Expressing Compassion . . . . . . . . 58

CHAPTER 5   **Celebrating Our Best**                                                          **63**

Positive Psychology . . . . . . . . . . . . . . . . . . . . . . . . . . . . . . . . . . . . . . . . . . . . . 63
How Does Coaching Generate Positivity? . . . . . . . . . . . . . . . . . . . . . . . . . . . . 64
Appreciative Inquiry (AI): A Tool for Celebrating the Best . . . . . . . . . . . . . . . . 65
But Really, What about Problem Solving? . . . . . . . . . . . . . . . . . . . . . . . . . . . . 72
Using Appreciative Inquiry to Transform the Coaching Relationship . . . . . . . . . 74

CHAPTER 6   **Harnessing Motivation to Build Self-Efficacy**                                  **77**

Harness Motivation to Build Self-Efficacy . . . . . . . . . . . . . . . . . . . . . . . . . . . . 77
What Does It Mean to Be Motivated? . . . . . . . . . . . . . . . . . . . . . . . . . . . . . . . 77
Motivational Interviewing: A Model for Increasing Motivation and Self-Efficacy . . . 80
Motivational Interviewing Principle 1: Engaging . . . . . . . . . . . . . . . . . . . . . . . . 80
Motivational Interviewing Principle 2: Focusing . . . . . . . . . . . . . . . . . . . . . . . . 82
Motivational Interviewing Principle 3: Evoking . . . . . . . . . . . . . . . . . . . . . . . . . 85
Motivational Interviewing Principle 4: Planning . . . . . . . . . . . . . . . . . . . . . . . . 86
Self-Efficacy . . . . . . . . . . . . . . . . . . . . . . . . . . . . . . . . . . . . . . . . . . . . . . . . . 86

CHAPTER 7   **Readiness to Change**                                                          **93**

Introduction to Change of Mindset and Behavior . . . . . . . . . . . . . . . . . . . . . . . 93
Transtheoretical Model of Change . . . . . . . . . . . . . . . . . . . . . . . . . . . . . . . . . 93
Stages of Change and Effective Coaching Skills for Each . . . . . . . . . . . . . . . . . 94
Supporting Clients in Moving through the Stages of Change . . . . . . . . . . . . . . 102
Readiness to Change Assessment . . . . . . . . . . . . . . . . . . . . . . . . . . . . . . . . . 104
Decisional Balance . . . . . . . . . . . . . . . . . . . . . . . . . . . . . . . . . . . . . . . . . . . 104
The Mount Lasting Change Model . . . . . . . . . . . . . . . . . . . . . . . . . . . . . . . . 106
General Suggestions for Coaching Change in Light of the Transtheoretical Model . . . 109

CHAPTER 8   **Client Assessment**                                                            **113**

The Value of Assessments . . . . . . . . . . . . . . . . . . . . . . . . . . . . . . . . . . . . . . 113
Assessments for Coaching . . . . . . . . . . . . . . . . . . . . . . . . . . . . . . . . . . . . . . 115
A Well-Being Assessment . . . . . . . . . . . . . . . . . . . . . . . . . . . . . . . . . . . . . . . 118
Coaching with a Well-Being Assessment . . . . . . . . . . . . . . . . . . . . . . . . . . . . 121

CHAPTER 9   **Design Thinking**                                                              **125**

Introduction to Planning . . . . . . . . . . . . . . . . . . . . . . . . . . . . . . . . . . . . . . . . 125
The Nature of Design Thinking . . . . . . . . . . . . . . . . . . . . . . . . . . . . . . . . . . . 125
Designing the Coaching Program . . . . . . . . . . . . . . . . . . . . . . . . . . . . . . . . . 126
Designing the Coaching Agreement . . . . . . . . . . . . . . . . . . . . . . . . . . . . . . . 126
Designing Visions . . . . . . . . . . . . . . . . . . . . . . . . . . . . . . . . . . . . . . . . . . . . 129
Making Visions Real: Designing Behavioral Goals . . . . . . . . . . . . . . . . . . . . . 132
Intermediate Behavioral Goals: The First Step in the Vision Quest . . . . . . . . . . 134
Designing Weekly Experiments . . . . . . . . . . . . . . . . . . . . . . . . . . . . . . . . . . . 134
The Role of Brainstorming in Goal Setting . . . . . . . . . . . . . . . . . . . . . . . . . . . 135
Tracking and Measuring Outcomes Progress . . . . . . . . . . . . . . . . . . . . . . . . . 137

Ask for Feedback on Coaching Sessions . . . . . . . . . . . . . . . . . . . . . . . . . . . . . . . . . . . . . . . . . 139
Putting It All Together . . . . . . . . . . . . . . . . . . . . . . . . . . . . . . . . . . . . . . . . . . . . . . . . . . . . . 139

CHAPTER 10    **Generative Moments**        **141**

Defining the Generative Moment. . . . . . . . . . . . . . . . . . . . . . . . . . . . . . . . . . . . . . . . . . . . . 141
When Do Generative Moments Occur within Coaching Sessions? . . . . . . . . . . . . . . . . . . 142
What Generates Generative Moments?. . . . . . . . . . . . . . . . . . . . . . . . . . . . . . . . . . . . . . . . . 143
Generative Moments Engage Every Coaching Skill . . . . . . . . . . . . . . . . . . . . . . . . . . . . . 143
Facilitating Generative Moments . . . . . . . . . . . . . . . . . . . . . . . . . . . . . . . . . . . . . . . . . . . . . 145
Relational Flow in Generative Moments. . . . . . . . . . . . . . . . . . . . . . . . . . . . . . . . . . . . . . . 151

CHAPTER 11    **Conducting Coaching Sessions**        **155**

Introduction. . . . . . . . . . . . . . . . . . . . . . . . . . . . . . . . . . . . . . . . . . . . . . . . . . . . . . . . . . . . . . . 155
Prepare for a Coaching Session. . . . . . . . . . . . . . . . . . . . . . . . . . . . . . . . . . . . . . . . . . . . . . . 156
Session Opening . . . . . . . . . . . . . . . . . . . . . . . . . . . . . . . . . . . . . . . . . . . . . . . . . . . . . . . . . . . 156
Goal/Experiment Review . . . . . . . . . . . . . . . . . . . . . . . . . . . . . . . . . . . . . . . . . . . . . . . . . . . 158
Generate New Learning with the Generative Moment . . . . . . . . . . . . . . . . . . . . . . . . . . . 162
Session Close . . . . . . . . . . . . . . . . . . . . . . . . . . . . . . . . . . . . . . . . . . . . . . . . . . . . . . . . . . . . . . 162
Handling Client Challenges . . . . . . . . . . . . . . . . . . . . . . . . . . . . . . . . . . . . . . . . . . . . . . . . . 162
Coaching Program Refresh or Close . . . . . . . . . . . . . . . . . . . . . . . . . . . . . . . . . . . . . . . . . . 164
APPENDIX A: Coaching Program Guidelines . . . . . . . . . . . . . . . . . . . . . . . . . . . . . . . . . . 165
APPENDIX B: Coaching Program Feedback Survey . . . . . . . . . . . . . . . . . . . . . . . . . . . . . 168

CHAPTER 12    **The Thriving Coach**        **173**

Last Words from Coach Meg. . . . . . . . . . . . . . . . . . . . . . . . . . . . . . . . . . . . . . . . . . . . . . . . . . 173
Human Thriving—Nine Primary Capacities . . . . . . . . . . . . . . . . . . . . . . . . . . . . . . . . . . . 174
The Call for Coaches. . . . . . . . . . . . . . . . . . . . . . . . . . . . . . . . . . . . . . . . . . . . . . . . . . . . . . . . 177

# CHAPTER 1

# Introduction

*"I saw an angel in the stone and carved to set it free."*

—MICHELANGELO

## Part 1—Defining the Role of a Coach

### OBJECTIVES

After reading Part 1 of this chapter, you will be able to:

- Define coaching and identify the value of the coach/client partnership
- Explain why professional coaches are needed to address health and wellness today
- Distinguish between the coaching approach and the expert approach
- Describe the current state of health and wellness coaching outcomes research
- Describe the coaching process

Welcome to the Wellcoaches *Coaching Psychology Manual*. This manual is designed to support education and training in basic coaching skills and processes. When we use the term "coach" throughout the manual, we are referring to professional coaches who work in health, wellness, and life domains related to well-being. The manual is of value to anyone interested in coaching knowledge and skills.

## What Is Coaching?

Coaching is a vehicle for helping people to achieve a higher level of well-being and performance in life and work, particularly when change is hard. Coaching is a growth-promoting relationship that elicits autonomous motivation, increases the capacity to change, and facilitates a change process through visioning, goal setting, and accountability, which at its best leads to sustainable change for the good.

The emerging industry of professional coaching, which began more than 25 years ago, focused initially on executive, business, and life coaching. Commercial and academic coach training and education programs have graduated more than 50,000 coaches worldwide. Health and wellness coach training programs emerged in the next stage, addressing mental and physical health and well-being in consumer, organizational, and healthcare settings.

Coaching is a partnership with clients in a thought-provoking and creative process that inspires and supports them to maximize their personal and professional potential, which is particularly important in today's uncertain, complex, and often overwhelming environment. Coaches honor the client as the expert in his or her life and work, and they believe every client has the potential to be creative and resourceful in order to fully self-actualize. Standing on this foundation, the coach's responsibility is to:

- Discover, clarify, and align with what the client wants to achieve
- Encourage client self-discovery
- Elicit collaborative and client-generated solutions and strategies
- Hold the client responsible and accountable (International Coach Federation [ICF], 2014)

Health and wellness coaches are professionals from diverse health and allied health backgrounds who work with individuals and groups in a client- (or patient-) centered process to facilitate and empower the client to achieve self-determined goals related to health and wellness. Successful coaching takes place when coaches apply clearly defined knowledge and skills so that clients mobilize internal strengths and external resources for sustainable change (National Consortium for the Credentialing of Health and Wellness Coaches, 2012).

Professional coaches in healthcare and wellness form partnerships with clients to optimize health and well-being by developing and sustaining healthful lifestyles. Coaches help clients enhance self-motivation and self-regulation, leverage strengths, navigate a journey of change, and build other psychological resources needed to change for good, including mindfulness, self-awareness, positivity, hope, optimism, self-efficacy, and resilience (Frates & Moore, 2011). Health and wellness coaches assist clients in connecting the dots between who they are and who they want to be, and in taking the incremental behavioral steps that will enable them to succeed in their desired changes, leading to a higher level of health and well-being.

Although some life and executive coaches may help their clients address health or wellness goals, they are typically focused on aligning personal and professional goals and values with improving well-being and performance in life and work. They don't have a primary focus on helping clients to establish health-promoting mental and physical behaviors that are aligned with evidence-based guidelines in fitness, nutrition, weight management, health risk, stress management, and life satisfaction.

Whatever the focus, masterful coaches use evocative, less frequently didactic, approaches with clients. They do more listening than talking, more asking than telling, and more reflecting than commenting. Coaching is not primarily advising clients on how to solve problems, simply educating clients about what they should do, nor analyzing the root causes of client predicaments. Although advising, educating, or analyzing problems are occasionally a part of coaching, they are not the primary purpose or approach of coaching. Coaches are collaborative and co-creative partners in clients' journeys to reach their visions and goals.

Coaches don't make it easy for clients by giving them answers; they facilitate the client's own self-discovery and forward momentum. Mastering health, wellness, and other life domains and developing the confidence to sustain one's well-being is a journey of personal growth. A coach is a partner in defining "Point B" and co-designing and co-navigating the journey to get there (Fig. 1.1).

The outcomes delivered by coaches include the following:

- Increased self-awareness and self-knowledge
- Increased personal responsibility
- Acquisition of new knowledge and skills
- Attainment of personal and professional goals
- Sustainable behavior change
- Increased life satisfaction
- Increased self-efficacy
- Developed sense of purpose and meaning
- Becoming one's best self

## Why We Need Health and Wellness Coaching

As it gains recognition over coming years, health and wellness coaching and wide dissemination of coaching skills have the potential to be a transformational force in the healthcare system in many countries. Coaching competencies can be applied in many settings (in-person and telephone, individual, and in groups) and by many professionals

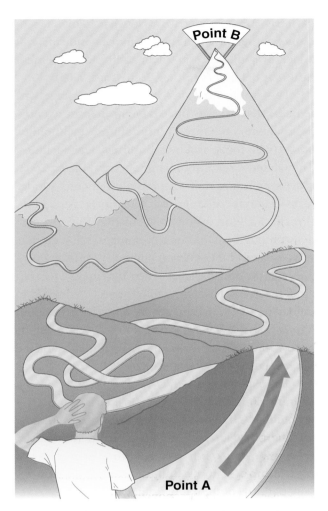

**Figure 1.1.** A coach supports clients in navigating from *Point A* to *Point B*, where they are to where they want to be.

(professional coaches, health professionals integrating coaching skills and tools into current protocols, and peer health and wellness coaches for community outreach). Coaches are focused on self-care reform (Gregory, 2013) as an important endeavor in the healthcare reform underway in many countries.

Lifestyle-related chronic diseases, heart disease, stroke, and cancer account for 50% of deaths, whereas obesity, prediabetes, and diabetes are reaching epidemic levels of prevalence in the United States and spreading globally. U.S. healthcare costs associated with lifestyle-related chronic diseases are estimated to be 75% of total costs (Centers for Disease Control and Prevention, 2013) and growing rapidly with an aging population engaged in unhealthy lifestyles.

Former U.S. Comptroller General David Walker (2012) notes: "Our current healthcare spending is unsustainable and could eventually bankrupt the country absent dramatic changes in our current healthcare programs and system."

Fewer than 5% (Berrigan, Dodd, Troiano, Krebs-Smith, & Barbash, 2003) of adults engage in the top health behaviors and only 20% of adults are thriving (Kobau, Sniezek, Zack, Lucas, & Burns, 2010). This is the first time in human history where being in control of one's health and making health investments day in and day out are poised to be dominant societal themes, just as smoking cessation was two decades ago, or sacrificing for the greater good was during World Wars I and II.

Health behaviors include stress management interventions as evidence mounts for the role of chronic negative emotions in impairing the brain's ability to learn and change in the present moment, and accelerating the onset of chronic diseases and early death (Cole, 2012). Meanwhile, mindfulness practices, which improve emotion regulation, have been shown to ameliorate a growing number of medical conditions (Marchand, 2012). Early research is showing that positive emotions and shared positive emotions in caring relationships improve mental and physical health (Fredrickson, 2013). A next research frontier is the role of meaning and higher purpose in improving well-being; published research by Cole and Fredrickson (2013) begins to suggest impairment of gene expression of the immune system in people with a low level of life purpose (Fredrickson et al., 2013).

The economic and clinical case for health-promoting behaviors as safe and effective interventions to help prevent and treat many chronic diseases is leading to a new medical domain—that of lifestyle medicine and the emergence of the American College of Lifestyle Medicine (www.lifestylemedicine.org) and the Institute of Lifestyle Medicine (www.instituteoflifestylemedicine.org) championed by organizations such as the American College of Preventative Medicine and the American College of Lifestyle Medicine. The second edition of a lifestyle medicine medical textbook was published in 2013 (Rippe, 2013) and included a chapter on health and wellness coaching (Frates & Moore, 2013), the first in a medical textbook.

Helping people take better care of their health is among society's most pressing priorities. In the United States, where employers assume a good deal of the responsibility for employee healthcare costs, organizational leaders are called upon to create workplaces that foster rather than damage health to both reduce healthcare costs and improve productivity and engagement (Moore & Jackson, 2014). Yet healthcare providers often do not have the skills nor are they reimbursed to help people learn and sustain new health-giving habits and leave behind health-damaging ones. The healthcare system was designed to manage acute medical emergencies and conditions. It is not well-suited to helping people manage a lifelong journey of developing and sustaining health-promoting behaviors. To date, a focus on prescriptive and expert educational approaches to helping people adopt health-promoting lifestyles has shown limited success (Frates & Moore, 2013).

Despite widespread knowledge about the serious risks of unhealthy lifestyles, many continue unhealthy habits or pursue quick fixes that don't last. Most people are not confident in their ability to lose weight or change their lifestyles. The demands of everyday life have never been greater. People face a bewildering array of health and wellness guidelines, products, and services, making it difficult to create a personal formula. Navigating the inevitable obstacles to making changes, including confusion, resistance, and ambivalence, is challenging. Many have histories of repeated failure. Most people do not believe they can reform their self-care or master their health and wellness.

People want to be well. They yearn to be in control of their health, to feel better, and to have more energy. But there is an enormous gap between wanting to be well and the everyday reality of living with the physical and mental health consequences of overeating, under-exercising, and having too little down time to recharge one's batteries.

New life skills are needed to develop a personal blueprint for well-being and become confident in one's ability to implement it. Most don't believe they are able to master these life skills. For example, the increasing numbers of those who choose bariatric surgery over lifestyle management techniques for healthy weight loss may be indicative of a lack of confidence in one's ability to implement healthier behaviors (Elfhag & Rössner, 2005).

The health and fitness industry is working hard to help. Never before have there been more experts, assessments, resources, guidelines, technology, books, web tools, and beautiful high-tech facilities. The wellness revolution is underway (Pilzer, 2002) with a welcome new emphasis on enabling long-term behavior change or "changing for good" (Prochaska, Norcross, & DiClemente, 1995).

Although all of these resources are valuable, more is needed. The "expert approach" of telling people what to do isn't ideal when they have low self-efficacy (Joos & Hickam, 1990). Experts are trained to deliver prescriptions and advice, and they often work harder than their clients in trying to help them. But the expert approach subtly lets the client or patient off the hook, sending the subtle message: *You are not in charge.*

The expert approach is vital when one is facing an immediate health crisis or considering surgery. It is not ideal when one wants to lose weight, reduce stress, or develop a positive and confident mindset. Delegating to experts comes with a price—loss of control and autonomy. Building confidence requires new patterns of thinking, doing, and relating.

The field of health and wellness also needs a shift in emphasis to strengths and opportunities, building on what's working and away from an emphasis on diagnosing and fixing what's not working. The more focus on the latter, the more self-confidence is undermined. It makes it harder, not easier, to change when the focus is on what's wrong and what's not working. Not enough positive energy and emotion are harvested to fuel the pursuit of change.

Moreover, clients need a whole-person view of health and well-being given our complex lives. Specialists who work in only one area, such as exercise, nutrition, or mental health without integration of the others, often experience a limit in their effectiveness. Multiple areas are intrinsically intertwined and are most successfully dealt with together. Most people need assistance with integrating information from multiple experts to decide what actions to take and how to prioritize them. People find it confusing when experts contradict each other. It is certainly not a recipe for promoting an "I can do it!" attitude.

In addition to unique genetics, each person is unique with respect to their history and preferences, diet trials and tribulations, and exercising or sedentary habits. More and more information on dietary allergies emphasizes the unique differences in our biology. People have their own food and exercise preferences. Some people love to jog and have been doing so since they were teenagers. Those same people are not necessarily swimmers. Other people love cycling or spinning. Disability or pain, such as knee pain from osteoarthritis, might limit the exercise options for some clients. Team sports such as basketball or soccer might be the best recommendation for an exercise routine. Zumba (a form of exercise dance which started in Latin America) has taken off among women as a fun, musical experience that doesn't feel like exercise. Preferences depend on the person, their past experiences, and their current interests and resources.

When it comes to providing information, different people have different learning styles. Some adults are visual learners who can benefit from graphs and pictures, whereas others are auditory learners who rely on lectures and conversations to consolidate information. Knowing your client and his or her learning style helps you adapt your approach so that your efforts will be effective and efficient.

It is important to approach each client as a unique individual, supporting his or her journey to find the formula which best fits his or her genetics, history, capacity, and way of life. Clients need to develop a wellness, health, and fitness habit portfolio that is tailored to their personal circumstances and capacities.

With a focus on building self-efficacy and autonomy, professional coaches are trained to:

- Accept and meet clients where they are today
- Ask clients to take charge
- Guide clients in doing the mindful thinking, feeling, and doing work that builds confidence
- Help clients define a higher purpose for health and well-being
- Uncover a client's natural impulse to be well
- Support clients in tapping into their innate fighting spirit

- Address mental and physical health together
- Assist clients to draw their own health and wellness blueprint
- Encourage clients to set and achieve realistic goals (small victories lay the foundation for self-efficacy)
- Harness the strengths needed to overcome our obstacles
- Reframe obstacles as opportunities to learn and grow
- Enable clients to build a support team
- Inspire and challenge clients to go beyond what they would do alone

## What Coaching Is Not: The Expert Approach

Coaching is an especially powerful methodology when it comes to stimulating individual behavior change because it is focused on helping clients grow into becoming more autonomous experts in their own well-being and personal path. Coaches first look to collaborate and partner rather than showing up as experts who primarily analyze problems, give advice, prescribe solutions, recommend goals, develop strategies, teach new skills, or provide education.

Although such expert approaches can be helpful in a coaching relationship, they are used "just in time" and infrequently. In the coach approach (Table 1.1), the client is called to become the decision-maker and to grow into the expert on the path forward as well as the evaluator of success. The goal of coaching is to encourage personal responsibility, reflective thinking, self-discovery, and self-efficacy. We want clients to discover their own answers and to create their own possibilities, as far as possible, rather than to be given answers or direction by the coach. Client-originated visions, plans, and behaviors are the ones that stick.

In 2010, Pollak and colleagues explored the impact on weight loss counseling when physicians were trained in motivational interviewing techniques. After one visit, the patients whose physicians used motivational interviewing techniques

| Table 1.1 | Comparing Approaches |
|---|---|
| **Expert Approach** | **Coach Approach** |
| Authority | Partner |
| Educator | Facilitator of change |
| Defines agenda | Elicits client's agenda |
| Feels responsible for client's health | Client is responsible for health |
| Solves problems | Fosters possibilities |
| Focuses on what's wrong | Focuses on what's right |
| Has the answers | Co-discovers the answers |
| Interrupts if off topic | Learns from client's story |
| Works harder than client | Client works as hard as coach |
| Wrestles with client | Dances with client |

Published in first edition. Created by Wellcoaches Corporation.

(collaboration, empathy, open inquiry, reflections) lost an average of 3.5 lb three months later. The patients whose physicians were not using motivational interviewing techniques gained or maintained weight. In just a few moments, coaches and healthcare providers can make a difference by using a collaborative rather than prescriptive dynamic.

Using the coach approach rather than the expert approach, coaches generally don't direct the client's goals and strategies, although they do guide the coaching process. They engage in coaching inquiries, asking powerful and insightful open-ended questions (what? how?) rather than closed-ended questions (do you? will you? did you?). They use reflections to mirror what they are hearing, such as, "You're feeling unhappy about your life balance, and you want to have more energy" or "You're excited and proud that you were able to walk three times this week, and it allowed you to time for peace and calm." And coaches listen, listen, and listen some more, with empathy and curiosity.

Coaches engage the minds and hearts of clients by assisting them in discovering their strengths, clarifying their values, increasing their awareness, setting their priorities, meeting their challenges, brainstorming possibilities, and designing positive actions.

Such engagement enables clients to generate a new self-concept (*Who is my best self?*), to create new supports and environments (*What supports my best self?*), and to take new actions (*What manifests my best self?*). By empowering clients to find their own answers, through asking nonjudgmental and provocative questions and delivering powerful reflections, coaches become catalysts for lasting change.

In transitioning from the expert to the coach approach, many coaches report the challenges as well as the rewards of:

- Asking questions with a beginner's mind—not assuming that they already know the answers
- Not making decisions and judgment calls quickly, but allowing clients the chance to go deeper and get to important topics
- Not thinking about what to say next, but instead listening for a dangling thread hanging off of a client's last words
- Not generating quiet resistance with even a hint of know-it-all energy
- Reading, respecting, and working with clients' emotions as possible guideposts to insights
- Not rushing clients through their "muck," but instead compassionately helping them sit there until the desire to change gains energy
- Not being on "automatic pilot" to ensure that a checklist gets completed, but instead being fully present to the client's reality and present needs

These and many other shifts can assist people with successfully mastering the health and wellness challenges of the present day. It can be especially difficult for healthcare professionals who have been trained extensively as experts and who are armed with large quantities of authoritative knowledge and written materials to support their expert status, to take off the expert hat, and shift to the coach approach. In many cases, it can also be difficult for clients to see and work with their coaches in a different way because they have long been conditioned to be told what to do rather than to take charge of their own health, wellness, and self-change. It is a challenge for coaches and clients alike to come from a new framework, but when the shift is made, the transformations follow.

Thomas Gordon (1970) has outlined twelve ways of being that do not demonstrate a coach approach:

1. Ordering, directing, or commanding
2. Warning, cautioning, or threatening
3. Giving advice, making suggestions, or providing solutions
4. Persuading with logic, arguing, or lecturing
5. Telling people what they should do; moralizing
6. Disagreeing, judging, criticizing, or blaming
7. Agreeing, approving, or praising
8. Shaming, ridiculing, or labeling
9. Interpreting or analyzing
10. Reassuring, sympathizing, or consoling
11. Questioning or probing
12. Withdrawing, distracting, humoring, or changing the subject

## Health and Wellness Coaching Research

The health and wellness coaching research literature while at an early stage, with studies trailing the latest developments in coaching education and skills training, is beginning to show that coaching interventions, multiple in-person or telephone coaching sessions for three months or longer, are improving health outcomes for several chronic diseases including diabetes, heart disease, obesity, and cancer survivors (Appel et al., 2011; Butterworth, Linden, McClay, & Leo, 2006; Edelman et al., 2006; Frates & Moore, 2011; Galantino et al., 2009; Newnham-Kanas, Morrow, & Irwin, 2011; Spence, Cavanagh, & Grant, 2008; Wennberg, Marr, Lang, O'Malley, & Bennett, 2010; Wolever et al., 2010). In 2013, Wolever and colleagues published a systematic review of the health and wellness coaching literature to identify 284 articles that operationalized health and wellness coaching:

1. A process that is fully or partially patient-centered
2. Includes patient-determined goals

3. Incorporates self-discovery and active learning processes (rather than more passive receipt of advice)
4. Encourages accountability for behavioral goals
5. Provides some type of education along with using coaching processes
6. Coaching occurs as an ongoing relationship with a coach who is trained in specific behavior change, communication, and motivational skill

Coaching competencies will continue to evolve as new discoveries are made by psychologists and neuroscientists. Coaching outcomes research addressing a wide spectrum of health and wellness needs from childhood to end of life is a vital endeavor to support the integration of coaching interventions into evidence-based medicine, healthcare, and consumer wellness offerings.

As is the case for any new professional domain, there is much progress to be made and research to be conducted to enable health and wellness coaching to become integrated into mainstream healthcare and corporate and consumer wellness. A U.S. volunteer organization, the National Consortium for Credentialing Health & Wellness Coaches (www.ncchwc.org) has developed standards, a national certification, as well as a collaborative research agenda to expand the evidence base. The Institute of Coaching at McLean Hospital, a Harvard Medical School affiliate, is awarding coaching research grants and furthering the translation of science into best coaching practices in healthcare and beyond.

## How Coaching Works

This manual describes the process of coaching as taught and implemented by Wellcoaches trained coaches and continually upgraded since 2002 and serves as an excellent starting point for new coaches or coaches who wish to expand their toolboxes. However, it is important to note that one cannot become a masterful coach by reading a manual. As in any skill-based work, the development of coaching skills requires practice, feedback, reflection, mentoring, supervision, and continued practice. This is why organizations such as the International Coach Federation (ICF), a coach credentialing and coach training program accreditation organization, and the Wellcoaches School of Coaching, a coach training organization, require mentoring and tests of a coach's practical application of skills to earn a coach certification.

## The Process of Coaching

Health and wellness coaches are not limited to helping clients improve diet and exercise. Health and wellness coaches address the whole person, what it means to thrive mentally and physically, and how to leverage the biology of change. The coaching relationship is designed to facilitate sustainable change and optimize health and well-being. With self-determination as a driver, clients move from dependency to empowerment, thereby making longer lasting, confidence-building, internally motivated changes that are appropriate for their evolving lives. Given that chronic stress directly damages health, the positive emotions generated by coaching will potentially be shown to reduce the incidence of disease symptoms, preventable chronic diseases, and early mortality.

In broad strokes, coaching progresses through several stages:

- Coaches and clients discuss a coaching contract so that clients understand the coaching process and expectations for the role of coach and client.
- Before and during the first coaching session, clients provide background information so that coaches are well-informed on the priorities, key concerns, and any medical conditions. Increasing self-awareness is an important goal of coaching, and assessments are an efficient tool to support self-discovery in the beginning.
- During the first coaching sessions (which may occur in one longer session or over the course of several sessions), clients work toward the creation of a vision, and three-month plan and goals to move toward a vision. Clients confirm that they are ready and want to do the work to make changes in at least one area. This is

also described as a wellness vision process and ideally is completed once per year.
- The vision and three-month goals are reviewed and agreed in detail. Clients also commit to three to five goals or small steps or experiments each week to enable progress toward the goals and vision.
- In each subsequent coaching session, weekly or as needed, coaches and clients review progress, elevating energy, brainstorming strategies, meeting challenges, developing solutions, generating possibilities, and agreeing on goals for the following week.
- During most sessions, a key topic is explored and resolved in a "generative moment" so that the client navigates around emerging challenges to continue on the change path.
- The ideal length of these sessions is 30–45 minutes, although some circumstances require more or less time. In fact, some protocols suggest that longer sessions (e.g., 60 minutes), occurring less frequently (once or twice a month) can have a greater impact than shorter, more frequent sessions. With the use of the coach approach, an impactful, life-giving, growth-promoting session is possible within even 10 minutes.

After a few weeks of coaching sessions, clients begin to notice some early wins and subsequent rewards, including improvements in how they feel and in their motivation to change. It's also not uncommon, after a burst of enthusiasm in the first few weeks, for clients to encounter challenges or setbacks. Both coaches and clients work hard to help clients engage their strengths, reignite motivation, find solutions, and brainstorm possibilities for meeting these challenges to reach the goal of establishing new behaviors. Anticipating, welcoming, and overcoming such challenges is a critical part of mastering new behaviors. It is what turns challenges into learning experiences.

Coaching sessions can be done face to face or by telephone or video conferencing. Phone and video conferencing coaching has become increasingly popular, particularly in addressing the needs of larger or remote populations. Although there are obvious benefits to working with a coaching client in person, sometimes more can be accomplished in phone and video sessions than in face-to-face sessions because there are fewer distractions and the distance helps minimize the client's disruptive, negative self-talk relative to the presence of the coach. Additionally, distance live coaching sessions can be more cost-effective to implement (Wennberg et al., 2010).

## Integrating the Coach Approach

The following considerations can assist coaches in knowing whether a coaching relationship is functioning effectively:

1. Make sure clients are working at least as hard as you are.
2. Make sure clients are talking more than you are.
3. Make sure clients first try to find the answers for themselves.
4. Ask permission to give expert advice, if you think it might be beneficial, so that the client is still in control.
5. Brainstorm two to three choices with a client so that the client taps into his or her own creativity and is the informed decision maker.
6. Speak less, and speak simply—deliver only one question or reflection at a time.
7. At every turn in the coaching conversation, stop and consider how to use the coach approach (inquiry/reflections) with the client before offering an expert approach.
8. Balance questions with reflections so that clients don't feel like they are being interrogated.
9. Use silence to elicit deeper thinking.

10. If clients confirm that they need to acquire new knowledge and skills to reach their goals and visions, help clients define the path to gaining the new knowledge and skills, with input from other experts when needed.

"Less is more" is a good rule of thumb for coaches when it comes to teaching, advising, and educating.

## COACHING CASE

**Example #1:** Wendy Well hangs up the phone and reflects on her coaching session with Coach Carl. Wendy recalls all of the insightful questions that Carl used. She wonders how he got to be so intuitive that he just knows what she is thinking without even having to say it. She is grateful that he is so wise and able to create great learning moments for her to move forward toward her goals. "Carl is a good coach," Wendy thinks as she smiles.

**Example #2:** Wendy Well hangs up the phone and reflects on her coaching session with Coach Carl. Wendy recalls all of the insights she had during the conversation. She tapped into her intuition and said things about herself that hadn't been said out loud until now. She is feeling wiser and is discovering new ways to move forward toward her goals. "I'm doing great!" Wendy thinks as she smiles.

In the second example, the coach has collaborated with the client in a way that builds her self-efficacy, confidence, and creative capacity for insight.

## Appendix A:

# What Brings Clients to Coaching?

Although people come to coaching for their own unique reasons, 12 themes are commonly cited by clients when they make the decision to invest in working with a professional coach:

1. Quick fixes over—"I'm done with quick fixes and want to make changes that last."

2. Precious asset—"I have decided that my well-being is my most precious asset, and I'm ready to invest for the long term."

3. Get off the fence—"I am fed up with sitting on a fence and want to commit to a wellness path."

4. Not about weight—"I realize that it's about well-being and not weight."

5. Be the boss—"I want to be the boss of my health and wellness and quit delegating responsibility to others."

6. Health style—"I'd like to develop my unique style of health rather than use one-size-fits-all approaches."

7. Mental game—"I know what to do and now want to master the mental game, turning intention into reality."

8. Peak performance—"I recognize that to reach peak performance at home and work, I need peak wellness."

9. Big picture/small steps—"I know that an extreme makeover isn't the answer, and I want to take small steps which are powerful."

10. Confidence—"I'm finished with self-doubt and want to build confidence in my ability to master wellness."

11. Winning the wellness game—"I want to focus on winning the wellness game and not losing or quitting."

12. Close the gap—"I want to close the gap between where I am and where I want to be when it comes to my health and well-being."

# Part 2—Coaching Psychology

## OBJECTIVES

After reading Part 2 of this chapter, you will be able to:

- Name the key components that make up the emerging field of coaching psychology, including the role of neuroscience
- Describe self-determination in theory and why it is a key theory in coaching psychology
- Describe four proposed coaching mechanisms of action

## What Is Coaching Psychology?

The first coaching psychologist, Anthony Grant (2011) at the University of Sydney, proposes a working definition of coaching psychology drawing on previous definitions proposed by the Australian Psychological Society and the British Psychological Society:

> Coaching psychology is a branch of psychology that is concerned with the systematic application of the behavioral science of psychology to the enhancement of life experience, work performance and wellbeing for individuals, groups and organizations. Coaching psychology focuses on facilitating goal attainment and on enhancing the personal and professional growth and development of clients in personal life and in work domains. It is not aimed at directly treating clinically significant mental illness issues or abnormal levels of distress. (pp. 84–99)

Coaching psychology, which can also be called coaching science, or the science of coaching relationships that are designed to deliver self-actualization, is vibrant, creative, and evolving rapidly. Today, coaching psychology integrates dozens of theories and academic fields, most recently the neuroscience field. It is being built by psychologists and coaching scholar-practitioners around the world.

Bodies of knowledge that are applied in coaching psychology include self-determination (Deci &

Ryan, 1985); positive psychology (Peterson, 2006); appreciative inquiry (Cooperrider & Whitney, 2005); nonviolent communication (Rosenberg, 2005); motivational interviewing (Miller & Rollnick, 2012); emotional intelligence (Goleman, 1996); design thinking (Brown, 2009); flow theory (Csikszentmihalyi, 1990); social cognitive theory (Bandura, 2001); adult and constructive development (Kegan & Lahey, 2009); and a number of therapy practices adapted to coaching such as cognitive behavioral therapy (Burns, 1980). Many of these bodies of knowledge are translated in this manual into coaching skills and knowledge to enable coaches to assist clients to learn, grow, and move forward in the direction of their desired goals.

## Self-Determination: The End Game of Coaching

The most respected theory of human motivation today, which also addresses primary human needs and well-being, is self-determination theory developed by Edward Deci and Richard Ryan at the University of Rochester over the past 30 years. The end game of coaching is self-determination—a client's ability to reach his or her highest level of motivation, engagement, performance, persistence, and creativity (Deci & Ryan, 1985). Ryan and Deci believe that to the extent that a coaching client's environment nurtures and meets three primary psychological needs (autonomy, competence, relatedness), autonomous self-regulation of behavior can occur. The need to feel autonomous (rather than controlled), the need to feel competent (confident and effective), and the need to feel related (having social support and connection that are autonomy-supporting) are addressed by coaches as resources for the journey toward higher self-determination.

According to Deci and Ryan (1985), three dimensions of the social environment can facilitate autonomy, competence, and relatedness. All of these dimensions are contained in the coaching relationship. The first is structure, which involves developing clear, realistic expectations; achievable goals; and encouraging capability as well as providing positive feedback, autonomy support, and involvement. It is important to note that the support of autonomy (self-determination), as well as of competence, is vital to fuel motivation. As a result of goal attainment, the client gains increased self-efficacy, a sense of autonomy and self-determination. According to Bandura (1997), self-efficacy beliefs come from performance experiences, vicarious experiences, imagined experiences, verbal persuasion, and physiological and emotional states. Self-efficacy is not only essential to our psychological well-being and physical health but also to self-regulation—how we guide our behavior in the pursuit of desired goals.

The second dimension is autonomy support, which involves acknowledging that clients have choices regarding behavior. This can be accomplished by encouraging a client to identify the purpose for a behavior, minimizing external rewards and punishments, providing opportunities for both participation and choice, and acknowledging whatever negative feelings are evoked when engaging in behaviors. To support a client's autonomy, a coach encourages the client to initiate behaviors based on a client's own values and desires, not those imposed by an external source such as a spouse, employer, or society as a whole. Owning one's reasons to change leads to greater autonomy and success. There has been much research showing that more autonomously regulated behaviors are more stable, leading to greater positive outcomes.

The third dimension, involvement, concerns the quality of relationships and the perception that significant others are invested, understand the person's challenges, and can reliably serve as psychological and emotional resources. Professional coaches serve as masterful supporters of client autonomy and self-determination.

## What Comes of Self-Determination?

A client who is experiencing high, autonomous motivation is more likely to have:

- Greater persistence
- More flexibility and creativity
- Better heuristic performance
- More interest and enjoyment
- Better mental health and well-being
- Better physical health
- Higher quality of close personal relationships

These findings are consistent no matter what age, socioeconomic status, and culture (Ryan, 2013). The bottom line—human beings are wired to thrive when granted the opportunity to engage in behavior that is of personal interest and value, when they are able to have a sense of competence around the behavior, and when they feel cared for and connected to other human beings on the journey to self-determination.

## Four Coaching Mechanisms of Action

Health and wellness coaches apply four coaching mechanisms to enable sustained change, a biological transformation of mindset and behavior. The first mechanism relates to designing a relationship that fosters brain learning, growth, and change. The second and third mechanisms can be considered the twin engines of change, also central themes in self-determination theory and motivational interviewing. People need to want to change, so they need to be motivated, and it has to come from within themselves. The second twin engine is confidence. They need to believe they can do it, feeling both "I want it" and "I can." Both need to be recharged frequently, even daily, to propel people forward. The last mechanism is the change process or journey itself, including assessments, visions, action plans, creative brainstorming, accountability, and referrals.

## Mechanism 1: Growth-Promoting Relationships

Drawing on humanistic psychology (Stober, 2006), coaches adopt the strengths-based stance that clients are not broken and needing to be fixed, but that they have the potential to be creative, resourceful, and resilient and are able to gain control and optimize health, well-being, and performance in life and work. Clients are too often focused on what's wrong, and they are out of touch with their full capacities.

Skilled coaches help clients figure out what they want and need, helping them find their own way, given a safe, nonjudgmental, challenging, and invigorating space. Aligned with Michelangelo's quotation, along the lines of "I saw an angel in the stone and carved to set it free," coaches help clients chip away at layers of life's clutter to reveal their best selves. Valuing the client's learning process more than they value their own expert knowledge, coaches help clients broaden and build on their strengths. Coaches know that they don't know many of the answers, and they hold a curious beginner's mind.

## How Coaches Help Clients Change Their Brains

Coaches support clients in developing new behaviors and mindsets by facilitating client-directed neuroplasticity over time, fostering the ideal conditions for a client's brain to change. Neuroplasticity is the brain's ability to grow, adapt, and change. Rewiring the brain is the process that underlies biological self-determination or self-directed neuroplasticity. The physiological mechanism for change is generally understood as the process of neurons forging new connections, creating new pathways and networks in the brain (Hammerness & Moore, 2012). Robust neural networks that endure likely require months, or a year or more, of client-directed neuroplasticity.

A coach's mindful presence is an important precondition to helping a client become mindful during a coaching conversation and encourages more mindful moments in a client's everyday life to improve self-reflection, self-awareness, self-regulation, self-compassion, positivity, and creativity, all noted below as critical to the brain's change process. Enhanced mindfulness enables coaches to improve listening skills; for example, being more present and not distracted by thinking about what to say next. A mindful state helps a coach better sense a client's positive and negative emotions, important messengers for both client and coach.

Coaching conversations help clients focus the brain's attentional resources on their personal ambitions and growth, enhancing the brain's ability to learn. A full focus of the brain's attentional resources is a first step in neuroplasticity and difficult to experience given today's epidemic of distractions. Undistracted attention, a state of full awareness, enhances neuronal activity by harnessing various regions of the brain, including the prefrontal cortex and subcortical limbic and brain stem areas, into an integrated coherent state. Attention enhances the responses of selected neurons under focus and reduces neural activity in other brain regions. An attentive brain can focus and learn without distractions, be productive and creative, and make fewer errors (Hammerness & Moore, 2012).

At its essence, coaching is a creative process, helping clients create neuronal connections and networks, imagine new possibilities, and develop new behaviors and mindsets. Carson (2010) has identified seven brain activation states or "brainsets" that enable the creative process, starting with a mindful absorbing of new information, intense reasoning or thinking about a problem to solve, envisioning or imagining a possible outcome, brainstorming to generate new possibilities, a flow state that produces a creative outcome, and an evaluation phase to enable sifting through options and implementing an action plan.

The brain is a connection machine, constantly making connections to reflect conclusions about how everything fits together, to make meaning of "it all" (Kegan, 1983). We are constantly trying to interpret the meaning of what happens to us, what others do, and what the effects are. Most activity in the brain involves creating connections between existing neurons and pruning these connections. Every piece of data, each idea, habit, and thought is made up of a set of connections among neurons. Making new connections and discovering new ideas and perspectives is pleasurable. When we create a new connection, we experience a positive charge of energy—the *ah-ha* of insight, temporarily opening our minds to new possibilities. A client's self-generated insights are important in supporting neuroplasticity.

Coaching sessions explore and make meaning of a client's values, vision, health, way of life and learning, challenges, and experiences along the journey of change. Clients move an automatic pilot mode of living into the spotlight of awareness and thoughtful reflection, and they take their personal relationship with health to a higher level of evolution. Instead of sacrificing thriving to meet life's demands, thriving becomes essential to meeting those demands. The meaning of health and thriving and one's ability to change the course of a way of life has changed for good.

A coach's skills engage, arouse, energize, and challenge clients to do the work needed to change their brains. They include not only "doing" skills such as listening, curious and open inquiry, and perceptive reflections but also "being" skills such as mindfulness, empathy, authenticity, affirmation, courage, zest, calm, playfulness, and warmth. Taken together, these skills enable coaches to build and sustain a close relationship and partnership with clients and promote brain learning and growth.

## Mechanism 2: Elicit Self-Motivation

There are two general categories of motivation—external and autonomous—as defined by Deci and Ryan (2002). Then, there are two types of external motivation. External motivation, or external regulation, occurs when someone other than ourselves, such as a boss, spouse, or parent, tells us what to do, and we don't think much about it beyond "I want to do what this person wants me to do to avoid conflict." For example, a coaching client might say "I'm exercising because my wife will get upset if I don't." That is the extent of his exploration and reflection. A second form of external motivation is when we internalize the external ideal, without a deeper alignment with personal values and desires, as an inner critic that says, "I should" or "I ought" to exercise or eat better. Although external motivation may work in the short term, it is not an effective form of motivation for the long term.

Autonomous motivation on the other hand does lead to sustainable motivation. Autonomous motivation often has a future orientation, for example, when we want to be fit and strong because we want to have the energy to make a difference every day or because we don't want our children to have to take care of us if we have a heart attack or stroke. Connecting a behavior to something in the future that we value, or the identity we want to project, is the type of motivation that has been shown to lead to sustainable weight loss. Then we have internalized our reason to do something because it is good for our future or fits with the identity to which we aspire. Future-oriented and desired identity-oriented autonomous motivation is the kind of motivation that works best (Deci & Ryan, 2002).

The other type of autonomous motivation that is also valuable is the one that produces flow experiences in our lives. It happens when we love to do an activity in the moment—we just love our yoga class, we are excited about cooking a new recipe, or we can't wait to listen to music to relax. When we love to do something, we do it for its own sake. We do it because it taps into our strengths, and it is fun and engaging. Although that can be a powerful kind of motivation for health behaviors, it can take many years to find. We may never fall in love with exercising, cooking, or meditation. It is important to keep looking, but it may not come along quickly. Clients need support in developing future-oriented, positive identity-based autonomous motivation, digging deeper to get to the "why behind the why." A client who wants to lose weight may initially be focused on wearing smaller sized clothes for a family celebration in a few months, and a coach may need to deepen the inquiry until a client has tapped into longer lasting, more meaningful motivation that will keep her on track while making dozens of health decisions each day. An example could be a heartfelt desire to be stronger and more energetic so as to not be physically dependent on her grown children as she ages, as she has watched her mother become.

Self-motivation is tapping into an energy source or a life force that is intrinsic and biological. It is often a heartfelt drive to help others, be a role model, make a difference in the world, to use our strengths competently, and to make our lives meaningful. Authentic motivation improves cognitive function, attention, emotion regulation, and creativity, bringing meaningful and dependable intentions to a challenging journey of change.

## Mechanism 3: Build Confidence

Although a high level of autonomous motivation is important to starting and sustaining a change journey, it is insufficient in the absence of self-efficacy or confidence in the face of one's obstacles. Capacity and confidence to change are typically built by diligent efforts over time. People have varying levels of self-motivation and confidence across a diverse set of eating, exercise, mindfulness, or emotional and self-regulation behaviors. If a client is reasonably confident and motivated to make even a small change, the success that follows will increase confidence and motivation further. Hence, it is often important to help clients select a habit that, while a stretch, is within reach and will build confidence a little. A little success will improve motivation and confidence and get clients started on an upward spiral.

Most people who have struggled with weight loss or a chronic disease for some time face many challenges that have led to failed change attempts and are stuck in a state called chronic contemplation. Self-efficacy is at a low level (Moore, Tschannen-Moran, Drake, Campone, & Kauffman, 2005). Cohen et al. (2009) has shown that not only do positive emotions allow us to be more open-minded and creative but they are also a main variable in determining one's resilience to setbacks and adversity. Ideally, each coaching session elicits and leverages a good dose of positive emotions. "What's the best thing that happened to you in the past week? What are you enjoying most in your life right now? What's your favorite thing to do? What makes you thrive or your eyes light up?" Coaches find ways to spark authentic positivity as a resource for creative brainstorming to bounce back from setbacks or circumvent challenges. Then, when clients inevitably reach

a roadblock, they can access more energy and creativity, improving the capacity to find new paths to rise above obstacles.

Another important approach to improving confidence is to help clients tap into another drive in Deci and Ryan's (2002) self-determination theory—to be competent. People dislike being incompetent; we hate falling off our metaphorical bikes, especially as adults. People are more competent and successful when they apply their values, strengths, and talents, as learned from the research in the application of character strengths (Niemiec, Rashid, Linkins, Green, & Mayerson, 2013). When clients tap into their strengths in new and creative ways, their mental processing comes up with solutions more quickly.

The Transtheoretical Model of Change (Prochaska, 1995) delivers tools to coaches that help clients determine client readiness for change of a given behavior, which is related to the level of self-efficacy. The model categorizes stage of readiness to engage in a behavior and then measures the use of key variables that have been found to promote behavior change. The four key variables are (a) stage of change, (b) decisional balance, (c) self-efficacy (i.e., examining challenging situations to create a personal relapse prevention plan), and (d) processes of change. Most recently, Norcross (2012) has translated the Transtheoretical Model of Change into a set of evidence-based emotional and behavioral processes that fit each of five stages of change: psych (getting psyched), prep (getting prepared), perspire (take action), persevere (manage slips), and persist (maintain change).

Along the journey, coaches help clients deal with setbacks in order to fully harvest learning. Creative brainstorming or relational flow is common in most sessions in order to generate new insights and increase hope and optimism by coming up with creative possibilities to navigate around numerable challenges.

## Mechanism 4: Process of Change

Just as organizations inch forward via projects that have strategies, goals, plans, and timelines, coaching clients focused on health goals benefit from structured projects and processes. Coaching often starts with health and wellness or well-being assessments to support progress tracking. Then, just like an architect creates a picture of a new house, the brain needs a vision or picture of what the ideal future looks like, the "envision brainset" in Carson's model of creativity (Carson, 2010). Next, it is time to design experiments, goals, and action plans that are set in motion to move clients toward their visions. Some clients prefer small steps, whereas others want the challenge of bolder goals.

Behavioral or SMART (an acronym for specific, measurable, actionable, realistic, and time-bound) goals, such as "I will do three 30-minute yoga sessions per week," focus on engaging in new habits consistently and provide specific ways to measure the success of goals. Clients may decide to set skill-building goals such as learning how to lift weights safely, cook healthy meals, or meditate, or they may want to set "performance" goals, such as reaching a certain weight or blood pressure level or completing a walking race.

Having clients determine how they want to be accountable is a critical step, as accountability to others is an important source of support. There are many mobile technology tools for tracking and accountability to self and others. Coaching organizations may provide online client files including assessments, tracking, goals records, and journaling. The simplest approach is a regular progress report, perhaps weekly, monthly, or quarterly. Setting quarterly or annual milestones for review and celebration provide important validation of progress. Clients may also need the support of other health experts and therapists along the journey, and coaches need to have a wide network of referrals and credible information sources at their fingertips.

It is important to note that coaching programs and sessions may have a structure, but coaching is not about following a formula. The peak moments of generativity, the heart of coaching sessions, are often described as an intuitive dance or relational flow (Moore, Tschannen-Moran, Drake, Campone, & Kauffman, 2005). In moments of relational flow, both coach and client are highly engaged, awake, challenged, and stretched to the outer edges of their abilities. During relational flow, clients shift perspectives and gain insights and new ideas. Clients change in these moments, and small forward leaps occur, which accumulate over time to lead to lasting change. These powerful coaching moments engage a coach's life force, too; delivering a growth-promoting partnership is one of life's greatest pleasures for coaches.

# Part 3—Training, Scope of Practice, and Professional Guidelines

## OBJECTIVES

**After reading Part 3 of this chapter, you will be able to:**

- Describe important considerations for coach training, self-care, and professional development
- Distinguish coaching and therapy
- Distinguish coaching and other professional roles
- Define liability and scope of practice guidelines
- Outline the ethical expectations for coaches.

## Becoming a Coach

Although the mastery of health and wellness and the life domains which impact mental and physical thriving are among one's highest priorities, most would agree that managing these are among the greatest life challenges, especially today when the environment is stacked against us. Supporting those whose spirits are buried under significant excess weight, those who haven't moved their bodies with vigor for a long time, or those who are "stressed out" is perhaps the toughest arena the world of professional coaching faces today. It is wise then for coaches to seek out the best training available. This manual helps set the bar.

Authentic empathy and complete acceptance come out of the pores of masterful coaches. They cannot summon an ounce of judgment. They have an uncanny ability to sniff out client strengths, values, and desires. They prefer to listen rather than talk. They love and enjoy client stories. They see the funny side in ways that facilitate growth. They hold up the mirror with courage when necessary. They have the patience to allow clients to sit in the muck, even in tears, without succumbing to the urge to rescue. They assist clients to achieve more than they otherwise might on their own. Masterful coaches

take risks to challenge clients to reach higher at the right moment. They know that lives are at stake if clients don't take great care of themselves. Best of all, masterful coaches know how to celebrate client success.

## Learning to Be a Coach

It is important for credentialed health and allied health professionals who are performing the role of a health and wellness coach to be trained and certified in coaching competencies. By learning how to competently use coaching skills and processes, experienced health and allied health professionals can improve the impact and results of their roles in helping clients and patients improve their well-being.

Some people are natural-born coaches with amazing aptitude for empathy, inquiry, mindfulness, insight, or courage. Others have developed their coaching skills through life experience. Even the best talents, however, benefit from formal training, mentoring, and certification (followed by years of practice, more training, and more mentoring to improve mastery). Learning and growth for coaches never stop, just as the process doesn't stop for clients; it is a lifelong journey. The coach training industry has plenty of opportunity ahead in developing more masterful coaches who assist people in becoming masters of their own well-being and of their lives (Williams & Anderson, 2006).

The International Coach Federation is one resource for identifying accredited coach training programs covering diverse specialties and niches. Wellcoaches coach training programs are a top recommendation for coach training, for both health professionals focused on health and wellness and nonhealth professionals combining coaching with a domain expertise such as career, retirement, or financial planning. Most of all, when selecting a coach training program, consider choosing one that:

- Provides evidence-based competencies, skills, and tools grounded in well-respected theories regarding the psychology of change and well-being or thriving

- Acknowledges the value of positive psychology and other tools honoring one's strengths, values, and resources
- Encourages client autonomy, self-efficacy, and collaboration
- Requires live practice of newly acquired skills and feedback from master coaches and mentors
- Employs faculty with training and extensive experience as professional coaches and coach trainers

## Practicing to Be a Coach . . . and a Client

To be an effective coach, it is important to experience being a client. It helps coaches understand the change process a client goes through. It also allows the coach to personally experience the results that can occur from a coaching partnership. Qualified coaches can be found through the ICF or Wellcoaches, depending on the area of focus. Working with a mentor who may provide more advice and training than a coach and developing a buddy or peer coach relationship are other avenues to help one grow as a coach.

Secondly, as with any new skill set, practice is the only way to learn to ride the coaching bike. The most important step one can take throughout the learning journey is intensive practice of the new skills and ways of being—shifting from being an expert to being a facilitator. Early in the learning process, it is valuable to recruit three to five practice coaching clients. There is much to be gained from applying the new skills of coaching early and often to better understand what works best, which skills come most naturally and which skills will require the development of new coaching muscles.

## Create a Professional Development Plan

Being a great coach is a lifelong journey; the learning and professional growth never stops. It is extremely important to sustain a deliberate and organized effort to continue to develop and expand one's skills as a coach. One possible step is to create a professional development plan:

- Assess your coaching skills on a scale of 0–10 (review all manual chapters to identify the most important coaching skills for self-rating).
- Set up your intended outcomes—where you want to be in six months and one year. Choose a couple of skills to work on at a time in three-month increments. This helps you focus.
- Develop an action plan to get there—what you are going to do. Use books, peers, skill practice, role-plays, classes, conferences, etc. in your plan.
- Set up a review time and make revisions.
- Celebrate all of the good things in your coaching life as well as your milestones as a developing coach!

Note that this same process can be applied to assess the coaching process while working with a client. For example, at the end of a coaching session or client relationship, reflect on the following questions:

1.  What am I learning about myself and others in coaching?
2.  Am I modeling wellness? If not, how do I see my role as a coach?
3.  What ideas of mine are being challenged in the coaching process?
4.  What am I discovering about myself?
5.  What are my strengths and weaknesses in working with this client?
6.  What mindset works best for me to facilitate my coaching?
7.  What stops me from saying what wants to be said?
8.  What don't I understand about my client, and what does this show me about myself?
9.  In what ways am I flexible, rigid?
10. In what ways am I being supportive or critical?
11. What judgments am I making about my client's life?

12. What surprises me in coaching?
13. What did I learn about the coaching process?
14. What in coaching makes me the most uncomfortable?

## Self-Care for the Coach

Taking care of oneself on all levels, or self-care, is an important part of optimal wellness. In fact, mastery of wellness can be considered mastery of self-care. Self-care can be defined as a way of living that incorporates behaviors that enable one to maintain personal health and balance, replenish energy and motivation, and grow as a person.

We all know the importance of eating a healthy diet and engaging in regular physical activity. But self-care goes beyond these basics and can include the following activities and many more: improving your physical surroundings; developing a practice that exercises your mind and soul; balancing family, social, and work demands with time to unwind by spending time in nature; soaking in a hot bubble bath; watching a beautiful sunrise; and listening to one's favorite music.

Practicing self-care does not come easily to many people who work in the "helping professions" because they are so accustomed to taking care of everyone else. It may feel selfish to "put yourself first" and take care of one's own needs when so many other things demand your time, energy, and attention. However, nurturing the body, environment, relationships, and spirit is a vital part of maintaining good health and a vibrant life, and it is a key factor in having the strength and motivation to continue to give to others.

Burnout is a stress syndrome that is prevalent among those working in health and helping professions. It happens when people try to reach unrealistic goals and end up depleting their energy and losing touch with themselves and others in the process. Burnout mainly strikes highly committed, conscientious, hard-working people and can be experienced by those who care passionately about the work they do. Burnout is "the extinction of motivation or incentive, especially where one's devotion to a cause or relationship fails to produce the desired results" (Freudenberger & Richelson, 1980). Because burnout is a condition caused by good intentions, it is easy to see how preventing it is important for coaches.

## Modeling to Be a Coach

Coaches share the same journey as clients: we are all seeking to walk the talk and to thrive. As ICF-Master Certified Coach Jay Perry says, "Coaching is not a service profession, it is a modeling profession." Throughout this manual, we will focus on how to structure the coach-client relationship so that it generates life-changing movement, learning, and growth on the part of the client. That is the point of coaching—to assist clients to clarify and reach their goals and to enjoy developing and strengthening their true selves in the process. However, this takes more than just the masterful use of coaching techniques. It takes a presence, a way of being in the world and with clients, which brings out the best in people through the quality of the connection itself. It's not just what the coach *does*, but who the coach *is* that determines our effectiveness in coaching.

For health and wellness coaches to manifest this presence and to generate this quality of connection, they need to "be the change they seek." In other words, coaches need to model in their own lives the very attributes of health, fitness, and wellness that they assist their clients to create. That doesn't mean a coach has to be "perfect," but he or she clearly should be on the path to discovering his or her best self. The more coaches experiment with and put into practice the wisdom that is developed with clients, the more transformational their presence will be. Clients respect and are inspired by coaches who "walk the talk."

To put on the mantle of role model without being boastful, coaches need to take care of themselves on all levels—physically, emotionally, intellectually, socially, and spiritually. Clients draw on the energy of a coach who is masterful at self-care, experiencing greater movement and change than they otherwise might. The better coaches attend to their own needs, the better they can help clients to do the same.

## Distinguishing Coaching and Therapy

Coaching and therapy are synergistic and different interventions, although there is an overlap in the tools and skills used by coaches and therapists delivering solution-focused, positive, and future-oriented therapy models. At its simplest, coaches help clients who are not experiencing serious mental distress build a better future, whereas therapists generally work with clients in distress and help them heal small and large emotional traumas and/or manage mental health conditions and dysfunctional mental patterns. Therapists are licensed to treat diagnosable disorders based on the *Diagnostic and Statistical Manual of Mental Disorders*, 5th edition (*DSM-5*), which includes all currently recognized disorders in mental health. Coaches are not clinical diagnosticians, and coaches do not focus directly on improving a clinically diagnosed condition, although coaching programs have promise as an adjunct to mental health interventions.

It's important that coaches are vigilant in noticing issues that may require the support of a licensed mental health provider. Some of the more obvious reasons that coaches would refer to an equipped mental health provider are when a client (Meinke, 2007):

1. Is exhibiting a decline in his or her ability to experience pleasure and/or an increase in being sad, hopeless, and helpless
2. Has intrusive thoughts or is unable to concentrate or focus
3. Is unable to get to sleep or awakens during the night and is unable to get back to sleep or sleeps excessively
4. Has a change in appetite, whether a decrease or increase
5. Is feeling guilty because others have suffered or died

6. Has feelings of despair or hopelessness
7. Is being hyperalert and/or is excessively tired
8. Has increased irritability or outbursts of anger
9. Has impulsive and risk-taking behavior
10. Has thoughts of death and/or suicide

Additionally, it is important to look for the less obvious indicators of mental health concerns that extend beyond the realm of coaching. Notice if a client keeps making attempts to change their way of living but keeps holding themselves back with self-defeating behavior or if a client wants to process feelings repeatedly rather than moving forward toward learning and insight (Arloski, 2013).

## COACHING CASE

Wendy Well set a goal to have conversation with her supervisor about decreasing her workload three weeks ago. Each week, Coach Carl and Wendy have discussed this goal, and no progress has been made. Instead, Wendy continually expresses doubt in her ability to have this conversation and often refers to her childhood experiences when she was criticized by her parents for speaking up when she had a concern. Carl notices this rumination on a past experience and the need to process these childhood feelings and says, "I'm noticing that the topic of your parents and their influence on you has been a part of our session for the last three weeks. It seems there are feelings to be resolved here that go beyond the work that you and I can do together in coaching."

## Distinguishing Coaching from Other Professionals

Following are distinctions among a variety of professions that are similar yet distinct from coaching, as provided by ICF (2015) and the National Commission for Health Education Credentialing (2014):

**Consulting:** Individuals or organizations retain consultants for their expertise. Although consulting approaches vary widely, the assumption is the consultant will diagnose problems and prescribe and sometimes implement solutions. With coaching, the assumption is that it is ideal for individuals or teams to generate their own solutions with the coach supplying facilitation, supportive, discovery-based approaches and frameworks, several options, and expertise when needed.

**Mentoring:** A mentor is an expert who provides wisdom and guidance based on his or her own experience. Mentoring may include advising, counseling, and coaching. The coaching process does not focus primarily on advising, mentoring, or counseling. It focuses instead on individuals or groups and teams setting and reaching their own objectives.

**Training:** Training programs are based on objectives set out by the trainer or instructor. Although objectives are clarified in the coaching process, they are set by the individual or team being coached with facilitation provided by the coach. Training also assumes a structured learning path that coincides with an established curriculum. Coaching is less structured without a set curriculum.

**Education:** Educators, particularly health educators, work to encourage healthy lifestyles and wellness through educating individuals about behaviors that promote healthy living and prevent diseases and other health problems. They attempt to prevent illnesses by informing and educating individuals about health-related topics and the habits and behaviors necessary to avoid illness. Although coaches may provide education, it is combined with coaching in a thoughtful way that enables client autonomy and choice.

**Athletic development and personal training:** Although sports metaphors are often used, professional coaching is different from sports coaching. The athletic coach is often seen as an expert who guides and directs the behavior of individuals or teams based on his or her greater experience and knowledge. Professional coaches possess these qualities, but their experience and knowledge of the individual or team together determines the direction in a more co-creative, collaborative model. Additionally, professional coaching, unlike athletic development, does not focus on behaviors that are being executed poorly or incorrectly. Instead, the focus is on identifying opportunity for development and new goal achievement based on individual strengths and capabilities.

**Therapy:** Therapy deals with healing pain, dysfunction, and conflict within an individual or in relationships. The focus is often on resolving difficulties arising from the past that hamper an individual's emotional functioning in the present, improving overall psychological functioning, and dealing with the present in more emotionally healthy ways. Coaching, on the other hand, supports personal and professional growth based on self-initiated change in pursuit of specific actionable outcomes. These outcomes are linked to personal or professional success. Coaching is future-focused. Although positive feelings and emotions may be a natural outcome of coaching, the primary focus is on creating actionable strategies for achieving specific goals in one's work or personal life. The emphases in a coaching relationship are on action, accountability, and follow-through.

## Liability and Scope of Practice

The potential for negative impact a coach can have on a client's well-being is important to consider. A coach needs to set clear limitations around his or her scope of practice to minimize liability risks of advice that could be harmful to a client. A coach should provide expert advice and teaching only in the areas in which he or she has nationally recognized credentials and follow evidence-based guidelines. Every client should be informed of the scope of practice and of the expert knowledge as validated by respected credentials that a coach brings to the relationship. If a coach is working with paying clients, professional liability insurance is also critical.

It is also important for coaches to apply their expert knowledge and step in when clients are doing or planning to do things that will endanger their health, fitness, or wellness (such as over-exercising, exercising unsafely when injured, not following a physician's prescription, sharing medication, following an unhealthy diet, or remaining in a high-stress situation). It is also important for coaches to *not* give advice on areas outside their areas of evidence-based competence and professional expertise. Coaching is no place for amateur advice.

The professional coaching industry takes the matter of coaching ethics very seriously. The ICF's Code of Ethics in Appendix B outlines expectations around conflicts of interest, professional conduct with clients, and confidentiality.

The Board Certified Coach credential, offered through the Center for Credentialing and Education, requires adherence to an ethics policy, which includes an emphasis on working only within one's scope of expertise, requiring all applicants to recognize the limitations of coaching practice and qualifications and providing services only when qualified, to seek supervision from qualified professionals when necessary, to provide referrals when unable to provide appropriate assistance to a client as well as when terminating a service relationship, and to ensure that clients, sponsors, and colleagues under-

stand that coaching services are not counseling, therapy, or psychotherapy services, and avoid providing counseling, therapy, and psychotherapy (Center for Credentialing & Education Board of Directors, 2010).

Wellcoaches certified coaches are required to adhere to clear standards as outlined in the *Wellcoaches Certification Handbook*:

- As a certified coach, you may provide expert advice only in the areas where you have nationally recognized credentials.
- You will inform clients of your scope of credentials and expertise.
- Any existing professional, licensure, or certification affiliations that certified health and wellness coaches have with governmental, local, state, or national agencies or organizations will take precedence relative to any disciplinary matters that pertain to practice or professional conduct.
- Wellcoaches certified coaches shall be dedicated to providing competent and legally permissible services within the scope of practice of their respective certification. These services shall be provided with integrity, competence, diligence, and compassion.
- Wellcoaches certified coaches are truthful about their qualifications and the limitations of their expertise and provide services consistent with their competencies.

## Appendix B:
# The ICF Standards of Ethical Conduct (www.coachfederation.org)

**Preamble:** ICF Professional Coaches aspire to conduct themselves in a manner that reflects positively upon the coaching profession; are respectful of different approaches to coaching; and recognize that they are also bound by applicable laws and regulations.

**Section 1: Professional Conduct at Large**

As a coach:

1. I will not knowingly make any public statement that is untrue or misleading about what I offer as a coach or make false claims

in any written documents relating to the coaching profession or my credentials or the ICF.

2. I will accurately identify my coaching qualifications, expertise, experience, certifications, and ICF Credentials.

3. I will recognize and honor the efforts and contributions of others and not misrepresent them as my own. I understand that violating this standard may leave me subject to legal remedy by a third party.

4. I will at all times strive to recognize personal issues that may impair, conflict, or interfere with my coaching performance or my professional coaching relationships. Whenever the facts and circumstances necessitate, I will promptly seek professional assistance and determine the action to be taken, including whether it is appropriate to suspend or terminate my coaching relationship(s).

5. I will conduct myself in accordance with the ICF Code of Ethics in all coach training, coach mentoring, and coach supervisory activities.

6. I will conduct and report research with competence, honesty, and within recognized scientific standards and applicable subject guidelines. My research will be carried out with the necessary consent and approval of those involved and with an approach that will protect participants from any potential harm. All research efforts will be performed in a manner that complies with all the applicable laws of the country in which the research is conducted.

7. I will maintain, store, and dispose of any records created during my coaching business in a manner that promotes confidentiality, security, and privacy, and complies with any applicable laws and agreements.

8. I will use ICF Member contact information (e-mail addresses, telephone numbers, etc.) only in the manner and to the extent authorized by the ICF.

## Section 2: Conflicts of Interest

As a coach:

9. I will seek to avoid conflicts of interest and potential conflicts of interest and openly disclose any such conflicts. I will offer to remove myself when such a conflict arises.

10. I will disclose to my client and his or her sponsor all anticipated compensation from third parties that I may pay or receive for referrals of that client.

11. I will only barter for services, goods, or other non-monetary remuneration when it will not impair the coaching relationship.

12. I will not knowingly take any personal, professional, or monetary advantage or benefit of the coach-client relationship, except by a form of compensation as agreed in the agreement or contract.

## Section 3: Professional Conduct with Clients

As a coach:

13. I will not knowingly mislead or make false claims about what my client or sponsor will receive from the coaching process or from me as the coach.

14. I will not give my prospective clients or sponsors information or advice I know or believe to be misleading or false.

15. I will have clear agreements or contracts with my clients and sponsor(s). I will honor all agreements or contracts made in the context of professional coaching relationships.

16. I will carefully explain and strive to ensure that, prior to or at the initial meeting, my coaching client and sponsor(s) understand the nature of coaching, the nature and limits of confidentiality, financial arrangements, and any other terms of the coaching agreement or contract.

17. I will be responsible for setting clear, appropriate, and culturally sensitive boundaries that govern any physical contact I may have with my clients or sponsors.

18. I will not become sexually intimate with any of my current clients or sponsors.

19. I will respect the client's right to terminate the coaching relationship at any point during the process, subject to the provisions of the agreement or contract. I will be alert to indications that the client is no longer benefiting from our coaching relationship.

20. I will encourage the client or sponsor to make a change if I believe the client or sponsor would be better served by another coach or by another resource.

21. I will suggest my client seek the services of other professionals when deemed necessary or appropriate.

### Section 4: Confidentiality/Privacy

As a coach:

22. I will maintain the strictest levels of confidentiality with all client and sponsor information. I will have a clear agreement or contract before releasing information to another person, unless required by law.

23. I will have a clear agreement upon how coaching information will be exchanged among coach, client, and sponsor.

24. When acting as a trainer of student coaches, I will clarify confidentiality policies with the students.

25. I will have associated coaches and other persons whom I manage in service of my clients and their sponsors in a paid or volunteer capacity make clear agreements or contracts to adhere to the ICF Code of Ethics Part 2, Section 4: Confidentiality/Privacy standards and the entire ICF Code of Ethics to the extent applicable.

### The ICF Pledge of Ethics

As an ICF Professional Coach, I acknowledge and agree to honor my ethical and legal obligations to my coaching clients and sponsors, colleagues, and to the public at large. I pledge to comply with the ICF Code of Ethics and to practice these standards with those whom I coach. If I breach this Pledge of Ethics or any part of the ICF Code of Ethics, I agree that the ICF in its sole discretion may hold me accountable for so doing. I further agree that my accountability to the ICF for any breach may include sanctions, such as loss of my ICF Membership and/or my ICF Credentials.

*Approved by the Ethics and Standards Committee on October 30, 2008. Approved by the ICF Board of Directors on December 18, 2008.*

### References

Appel, L. J., Clark, J. M., Yeh, H. C., Wang, N. Y., Coughlin, J. W., Daumit, G., . . . Brancati, F. L. (2011). Comparative effectiveness of weight-loss interventions in clinical practice. *The New England Journal of Medicine, 365,* 1959–1968.

Arloski, M. (2013). *The wellness coach and referring clients to a mental health professional.* Retrieved May 3, 2015 from http://realbalancewellness.wordpress.com/2013/02/11/the-wellness-coach-and-referring-clients-to-a-mental-health-professional-part-one-when/

Bandura, A. (1997). *Self-efficacy: The exercise of control.* New York: W. H. Freeman.

Bandura, A. (2001). Social cognitive theory: An agentic perspective. *Annual Review of Psychology, 52,* 1–26.

Berrigan, D., Dodd, K., Troiano, R. P., Krebs-Smith, S. M., & Barbash, R. B. (2003). Patterns of health behavior in U.S. adults. *Preventive Medicine, 36*(5), 615–623.

Brown, T. (2009). *Change by design: How design thinking transforms organizations and inspires innovation.* New York: Harper Business.

Burns, D. D. (1980). *Feeling good: The new mood therapy.* New York: William Morrow.

Butterworth, S., Linden, A., McClay, W., & Leo, M. (2006). Effect of motivational interviewing-based health coaching on employees' physical and mental health status. *Journal of Occupational Health Psychology, 11*(4), 358–365.

Carson, S. (2010). *Your creative brain: seven steps to maximize imagination, productivity, and innovation in your life.* Boston: Harvard Health Publications.

Center for Credentialing & Education Board of Directors. (2010). *Board certified coach code of ethics.* Retrieved March 25, 2014 from http://www.cce-global.org/Downloads/Ethics/BCCcodeofethics.pdf

Centers for Disease Control and Prevention. (2013). *Chronic Diseases and Health Promotion.* Retrieved May 3, 2015 from http://www.cdc.gov/chronicdisease/overview/

Cohn, M. A., Fredrickson, B. L., Brown, S. L., Mikels, J. A., & Conway, A. M. (2009). Happiness unpacked:

Positive emotions increase life satisfaction by building resilience. *Emotion, 9*, 361–368.

Cole, S. (2012). Social regulation of gene expression in the immune system. In S. Segerstrom (Ed.), *Oxford handbook of psychoneuroimmunology* (pp. 254–273). New York: Oxford University Press.

Cooperrider, D., & Whitney, D. (2005). *Appreciative inquiry: A positive revolution in change.* San Francisco: Berrett-Koehler.

Csikszentmihalyi, M. (1990). *Flow.* New York: Harper & Row.

Deci, E. L., & Ryan, R. M. (1985). *Intrinsic motivation and self-determination in human behavior.* New York: Plenum Press.

Deci, E. D., & Ryan, R. M. (2002). *Handbook of self-determination research.* New York: University of Rochester Press.

Edelman, D., Oddone, E. Z., Liebowitz, R. S., Yancy, W. S., Jr., Olsen, M. K., Jeffreys, A. S., . . . Gaudet, T. W. (2006). A multidimensional integrative medicine intervention to improve cardiovascular risk. *Journal of General Internal Medicine, 21*(7), 728–734.

Elfhag, K., & Rössner, S. (2005). Who succeeds in maintaining weight loss? A conceptual review of factors associated with weight loss maintenance and weight regain. *Obesity Reviews, 6*(1), 67–85.

Frates, B., & Moore, M. (2011). Coaching for behavior change in physiatry. *American Journal of Physical Medicine & Rehabilitation, 90*(12), 1074–1082.

Frates, B., & Moore, M. (2013). Health and wellness coaching skills for lasting change. In J. M. Rippe (Ed.), *Lifestyle Medicine* (2nd ed., pp. 343–360). New York: CRC Press.

Fredrickson, B. (2013a). *Love 2.0: Creating happiness and health in moments of connection.* New York: Plume.

Fredrickson, B. (2013b). *Love 2.0.: How our supreme emotion affects everything we feel , think, do, and become.* New York: Hudson Street Press.

Fredrickson, B., Grewen, K. M., Coffey, K. A., Algoe, S. B., Firestine, A. M., Arevalo, J. M., . . . Cole, S.W. (2013). A functional genomic perspective on human well-being. *Proceedings of the National Academy of Sciences, 110*(33), 13684–13689.

Freudenberger, H., & Richelson, G. (1980). *Burnout: The high cost of achievement.* Garden City, NY: Anchor Press.

Galantino, M. L., Schmid, P., Milos, A., Leonard, S., Botis, S., Dagan, C., . . . Mao, J. (2009). Longitudinal benefits of wellness coaching interventions for cancer survivors. *International Journal of Interdisciplinary Social Sciences, 4*(10), 41–58.

Goleman, D. (1996). *Emotional intelligence.* New York: Bantam.

Gordon, T. (1970). *Parent effectiveness training.* New York: Wydenn.

Grant, A. (2011). Developing an agenda for teaching coaching psychology. *International Coaching Psychology Review, 6*(1), 84–99.

Gregory, R. (2013). *Self-care reform: How to discover your own path to good health.* Charleston, SC: CreateSpace Independent Publishing Platform.

Hammerness, P. & Moore, M. (2012). *Organize your mind, organize your life.* Harvard Health book. Ontario: Harlequin.

International Coach Federation. (2014). *Core competencies.* Retrieved May 3, 2015 from http://coachfederation.org/credential/landing.cfm?ItemNumber=2206&navItemNumber=576

International Coach Federation. (2015). *What is professional coaching?* Lexington, KY: Author. Retrieved May 3, 2015 from http://coachfederation.org/need/landing.cfm?ItemNumber=978&navItemNumber=567

Joos, S. K., & Hickam, D. H. (1990). How health professionals influence health behavior: Patient-provider interaction and health care outcomes. In K. Glans, F. M. Lewis, & B. K. Rimer (Eds.), *Health behavior and health education: Theory, research and practice* (pp. 216–241). San Francisco: Jossey-Bass.

Kegan, R. (1983). *The evolving self: Problem and process in human development.* Boston: Harvard Press.

Kegan, R., & Lahey, L. (2009). *Immunity to change: How to overcome it and unlock the potential in yourself and your organization.* Boston, MA: Harvard Business Review Press.

Kobau, R., Sniezek, J., Zack, M., Lucas, R., & Burns, A. (2010). Well-being assessment: An evaluation of well-being scales for public health and population estimates of well-being among US adults. *Applied Psychology: Health and Wellbeing, 2*(3), 272–297.

Marchand, W. (2012). Mindfulness-based stress reduction, mindfulness-based cognitive therapy, and Zen meditation for depression, anxiety, pain and psychological distress. *Journal of Psychiatric Practice, 18*(4), 233–252.

Meinke, L. (2007). *Top ten indicators to refer a client to a mental health professional.* Lexington, KY: International Coach Federation.

Miller, W. R., & Rollnick, S. (2012). *Motivational interviewing: Helping people change.* New York: Guildford Press.

Moore, M., & Jackson, E. (2014). Health and wellness coaching. In E. Cox, T. Bachkirove, & D. Ashley (Eds.),

*The complete handbook of coaching.* Thousand Oaks: SAGE Publications.

Moore, M., Tschannen-Moran, B., Drake, D., Campone, F., & Kauffman, C. (2005). Relational flow: A theoretical model of the intuitive dance of coaching. *Proceedings of the Third International Coach Federation Coaching Research Symposium.* Lexington, KY: International Coach Federation.

National Commission for Health Education Credentialing. (2014). *Responsibilities and competencies.* Retrieved May 3, 2015 from http://www.nchec.org/responsibilities-and-competencies

National Consortium for the Credentialing of Health and Wellness Coaches. Retrieved May 12, 2015 from www.ncchwc.org

Niemiec, R. M., Rashid, T., Linkins, M., Green, S., & Mayerson, N. H. (2013). Character strengths in practice. *IPPA Newsletter, 5*(4).

Newnham-Kanas, C., Morrow, D., & Irwin, J. (2011). Participants' perceived utility of motivational interviewing using Co-Active Life Coaching skills on their struggle with obesity. *Coaching: An International Journal of Theory, Research and Practice, 4*(2), 104–122.

Norcross, J. (2012). *Changeology: 5 steps to realizing your goals and resolutions.* New York: Simon and Schuster.

Peterson, C. (2006). *A primer in positive psychology.* New York: Oxford University Press.

Pilzer, P. Z. (2002). *The wellness revolution.* Hoboken, NJ: John Wiley & Sons.

Pollak, K. I., Alexander, S. C., Coffman, C. J., Tulsky J. A., Lyna, P., Dolor, R. J., . . . Østbye, T. (2010). Physician communication techniques and weight loss in adults: Project CHAT. *American Journal of Preventive Medicine, 39*(4), 321–328.

Prochaska, J., Norcross, J., & DiClemente, C. (1995). *Changing for good: A revolutionary six-stage program for overcoming bad habits and moving your life positively forward.* New York: William Morrow Paperbacks.

Prochaska, J. O., Norcross, J. C., & DiClemente, C. C. (1995). *Changing for good: A revolutionary six-stage program for overcoming bad habits and moving your life positively forward.* New York: Harper Collins.

Rippe, J. (2013). *Lifestyle medicine.* Boca Raton, FL: CRC Press.

Rosenberg, M. (2005). *Nonviolent communication: A language of life.* Encinitas, CA: PuddleDancer.

Ryan, R. (2013, September). *On motivating oneself and others: Research and interventions using self-determination theory.* Paper presented at Coaching in Leadership and Healthcare Conference 2013, Harvard/McLean Medical School, Cambridge, MA.

Ryan R. M., & Deci, E. L. (2002). Overview of self-determination theory: An organismic dialectal perspective. In E. L. Deci & R. M. Ryan (Eds.), *Handbook of self-determination research* (pp. 3–33). Rochester, NY: University of Rochester Press.

Spence, G. B., Cavanagh, M. J., & Grant, A. M. (2008). The integration of mindfulness training and health coaching: An exploratory study. *Coaching: An International Journal of Theory, Research and Practice, 1*(2), 1–19.

Stober, D. R. (2006). Coaching from a humanistic perspective. In D. R. Stober & A. M. Grant (Eds.), *Evidence based coaching handbook* (pp. 17–50). Hoboken, NJ: John Wiley & Sons.

Walker, D. (2012). Gambling with the future of healthcare. *Healthcare Finance.* Retrieved May 12, 2015 from http://www.healthcarefinancenews.com/news/gambling-future-healthcare

Wennberg, D., Marr, A., Lang, L., O'Malley, S., & Bennett, G. (2010). A randomized trial of telephone care-management strategy. *The New England Journal of Medicine, 363,* 1245–1255.

Williams, P., & Anderson, S. K. (2006). *Law & ethics in coaching: How to solve and avoid difficult problems in your practice.* Hoboken, NJ: John Wiley & Sons.

Wolever, R., Dreusicke, M., Fikkan, J., Hawkins, T. V., Yeung, S., Wakefield, J., Duda, L. . . . Skinner, E. (2010). Integrative health coaching for patients with type 2 diabetes. *The Diabetes Educator, 36*(4), 629–639.

Wolever, R., Simmons, L. A., Sforzo, G. A., Dill, D., Kaye, M., Bechard, E. M., . . . Yang, N. (2013). A systematic review of the literature on health and wellness coaching: Defining a key behavioral intervention in healthcare. *Global Advances in Health and Medicine, 2,* 38–57.

# CHAPTER 2

# Coaching Relationship Skills

*"The coach's certainty is greater than the client's doubt."*

—Dave Buck, President of CoachVille

## OBJECTIVES

**After reading this chapter, you will be able to:**

- Define the coaching relationship, the "heart of coaching"
- Describe the skills for establishing trust and building rapport within a coaching relationship
- Name and discuss three core coaching skills
- Identify the skills for mindful listening, open-ended inquiry, and perceptive reflections
- Identify additional tools for developing the coaching relationship
- Connect the building of strong relationships to self-determination theory

## Relationship: The Heart of Coaching and Growth

A trusting, authentic, and connected bond between coach and client is the first goal of any coaching relationship. The following summarizes the perspectives of a variety of expert coaches and coaching organizations who place high value on the coach-client relationship:

*"Coaching Mastery:* Establishing and maintaining a relationship of trust.

*Definition:* Ensure a safe space and supportive relationship for personal growth, discovery, and transformation.
*Effect:* The client is open to sharing and receiving; the client perceives the coach as a personal advocate; the client sees transformation and growth as manageable; and the client has realistic expectations of results and responsibilities of coaching.
*Key Elements:* Mutual respect and acceptance; confidence and reassurance; and the client feels safe to share fears without judgment from the coach."—International Association of Coaching, 2014

*"Coaching Competency:* Co-creating the Relationship
*How:* Establishing trust and intimacy with the client—ability to create a safe, supportive environment that produces ongoing mutual respect and trust.

- Shows genuine concern for the client's welfare and future
- Continuously demonstrates personal integrity, honesty and sincerity
- Establishes clear agreements and keeps promises
- Demonstrates respect for client's perceptions, learning style, personal being
- Provides ongoing support for and champions new behaviors and actions, including those involving risk taking and fear of failure
- Asks permission to coach client in sensitive, new areas"—International Coach Federation, 2014

"Coaching is that part of a relationship in which a person is primarily dedicated to serving the long-term development, competence, self-generation, and aliveness in the other."—Doug Silsbee, *Presence-Based Coaching,* 2008

"Coaching is the art of creating an environment through conversation and a way of being that facilitates the process by which a person can move toward desired goals in a fulfilling manner."—Tim Gallwey, *The Inner Game of Work,* 2000, p. 177

"Coaching is a process that fosters self-awareness and that results in the motivation to change as well as the guidance needed if change is to take place in ways that meet organizational performance needs."—David Dotlich and Peter Cairo, *Action Coaching,* 1999, p. 31

"Coaching is essentially a growth and results-oriented conversation—a dialog between a coach and a coachee. Coaching helps individuals access what they can discover given a deeply reflective and collaborative mindset. Clients may never have asked themselves the coach's questions, and they have a greater ability to discover answers than they often appreciate. A coach assists, supports, and encourages individuals to discover their answers. Coaching is about fostering learning—yet a coach is not a teacher and does not always know how to do things better than the client. A coach can notice and observe patterns, set a stage for new actions, and then work with a client to put these new, more successful actions into place.

Through various coaching techniques such as listening, reflecting, asking questions, and providing information, clients become more self-reflective, self-correcting, and self-generating. Coaching starts by asking the right questions—a coach engages in a collaborative alliance with the individual to establish and clarify purpose and goals and to develop a plan of action to achieve these goals."—Perry Zeus and Suzanne Skiffington, *The Complete Guide to Coaching at Work,* 2000, p. 3

Despite nuances of perspective and emphasis, these definitions of coaching share a common denominator: relationship. Human beings are fundamentally and pervasively motivated by a need to belong, by a strong desire to form and maintain enduring personal attachments; they seek frequent positive interaction within the context of long-term, caring relationships (Baumeister & Leary, 1995). Coaching is one such growth-fostering relationship that enables clients to reach their goals and get closer to their visions.

It has long been thought that the relationship between a helper (therapist or coach) and a client is the fundamental ingredient in positive outcomes. This was confirmed in a meta-analysis completed by Norcross and Lambert (2010), which found that the therapy relationship makes substantial and consistent contributions to patient success in all types of psychotherapy studied (e.g., psychodynamic, humanistic, cognitive, behavioral, systemic) and accounts for why clients improve (or fail to improve) as much as the particular treatment method (Norcross & Lambert, 2010). Based on coaching research, De Haan (2008) reports that the quality of the coach-client relationship (also called "working alliance") is the best predictor of client success. It's not that the client who experienced positive outcomes described the relationship as positive, but that a relationship deemed positive at the beginning of the engagement leads to subsequent positive outcomes. The second most important factor reported was a set of personal characteristics for the coach—being empathetic, inspiring confidence, appearing competent, his or her own positive mental health, and the ability of the coach to operate from the client's value system (Fig. 2.1) (De Haan, 2008).

The core coaching skills described in this chapter are also consistent with International Coach Federation's core coaching competencies (International Coach Federation, 2014) and the International Association of Coaching's list of coaching masteries

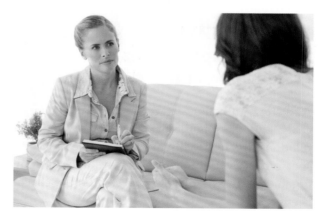

**Figure 2.1.** The success of the coaching experience depends on the coaching relationship.

(certifiedcoach.org) and are widely taught by coach education and training schools. These skills are not new discoveries by coaches; rather, they are foundational relational skills of counseling and clinical psychologists and are core skills of the motivational interviewing approach used both in therapy and in coaching.

Most importantly, a respectful, collaborative, client-centered coaching relationship also supports self-determination.

> "Many models of intervention and change have suggested that the practitioner-patient relationship is an important medium and vehicle of change. In healthcare this is especially so, as vulnerable individuals, often lacking in technical expertise, look for the inputs and guidance of professionals. In this process, a sense of being respected, understood, and cared for is essential to forming the experiences of connection and trust that allow for internalization to occur." (Ryan et al., 2008).

Relatedness, one of the key components in the development of self-determination, is nurtured when one is in a relationship; it conveys respect, and the individual feels valued and experiences warmth and empathy from the coach.

## Establishing Trust and Rapport

The coaching relationship requires the establishment of strong trust and rapport in order to generate a productive and fulfilling change process. When trust and rapport are absent, so is a growth-fostering environment. Megan Tschannen-Moran (2004) defines trust as the "willingness to be vulnerable to another based on the confidence that the other is benevolent, honest, open, reliable, and competent." Understanding the importance of these five qualities, masterful coaches pay constant attention to using them in every conversation. Additional dimensions of relationship building are expanded in the following.

## Hold Unconditional Positive Regard

According to Carl Rogers (1995), unconditional positive regard is defined as "being completely accepting toward another person, without reservations." Holding such regard for clients is essential for establishing rapport and trust. The coaching alliance will be weak and unsuccessful if clients do not believe that their coaches are on their side, accepting them unconditionally.

Judgment, criticism, and disappointment—both spoken and unspoken—do not motivate or support behavior change. It is not appropriate for the coach to point out clients' shortcomings and teach them better ways; rather, a coach is called to champion clients' strengths and invite them to figure out better ways. When a coach believes in his or her clients and holds positive regard for them—regardless of what they do or do not accomplish—the relationship can bolster both self-efficacy and self-esteem. Unfailing positive regard is the key to establishing rapport and trust, and it is the foundation for masterful coaching.

## Show Empathy

Traditionally, empathy is defined as "the feeling that you understand and share another person's experiences and emotions: the ability to share someone else's feelings." The difficulty with this view of empathy in the coaching relationship is that it can distract from the focus on the client's agenda and shift focus to the experience (feelings, perspectives, opinions) of the coach. This can lead to more undesirable attitudes such as sympathy (identifying with the client's experience on an emotional level and experiencing the same emotions or emotional contagion) and pity (a strong feeling of sadness or sympathy for someone or something that causes sadness or disappointment).

In the context of coaching, empathy is more accurately defined as a respectful understanding of another person's experience, including his or her feelings, needs, and desires. From this perspective, empathy is quite different from sympathy. Someone who is sympathetic identifies with another's experience, whereas an empathetic person seeks to understand and appreciate that experience. And empathy acknowledges the client's right to feel and experience the situation however he or she chooses without needing pity, sadness, or disappointment from the coach. Coaching is made possible by empathic engagement that builds relationships and facilitates growth.

Empathy helps build trust and rapport. When clients are struggling, it's especially important to connect with their feelings, needs, and desires in a positive, supportive, and understanding way. When clients feel judged, their self-efficacy and readiness to change may be undermined. When clients feel a lack of compassion, they may become resistant to coaching resources.

## Be a Humble Role Model

To develop trust and rapport with clients, coaches serve as humble role models for optimal health and wellness, "walking the talk" without being boastful, arrogant, or rude. Humility is present when a coach is continually working on his or her own fulfillment, balance, health, fitness, and well-being, knowing there is still much to learn. The challenge is to be a role model without placing oneself on a pedestal or talking too much about one's own successes. The key is to never dominate the conversation with one's own experiences in an eagerness to help and to always remain humble.

At the start of a coaching partnership, coaches typically deliver a brief yet inspirational introduction that captures our passion for health, fitness, wellness, and coaching. A succinct summary of a coach's background and how he or she works with clients should be included. "What more do you want to know about me?" is a great way to end the summary and invite questions that build rapport.

People come to coaching not only to learn, but also for inspiration. Most people already know or at least have a sense of what they "should" be doing to improve health, fitness, and wellness. They just don't know how to do it consistently. By drawing close to someone who does, like a coach, they hope to gain insight and inspiration for the journey. Personal disclosure on the part of the coach is appropriate and valuable when it serves the best interests of the client and the coaching program, not because a coach wants to share and be understood (subtly inviting the client to play the helper role). A coach

must carefully discern if and when to share who he or she is; why he or she cares about health, fitness, and wellness; how he or she lives; his or her victories and struggles; and what he or she knows and doesn't know about health and wellness.

## Slow Down

It is important to continue to establish trust and rapport in each and every coaching session. Trust and rapport are not earned in a single moment. They are earned or lost during every moment of coaching sessions. If coaches are in a hurry to "get down to business," trust and rapport will be compromised or lost. Coaches need to set aside the time to have a relaxed—and relaxing—presence with clients. Even when appointments are scheduled back to back, it is important to slow down, be completely present, and savor every moment with each client.

## Under-Promise and Over-Deliver

Nothing undermines trust and rapport more than broken promises. That is why it is extremely important to monitor and select one's words carefully, both during coaching sessions and in communications between sessions. A professional coach delivers on every promise. Some promises, such as being ready and available when clients call for coaching, are unspoken parts of the coaching agreement. Other promises, such as sending clients information, are offered in the course of conversation.

Delivering on all promises is crucial to the coaching relationship. Be careful to not fall into the trap of over-promising and under-delivering. This may be common in our society, as people seek to make themselves look good, but it quickly leads to failed coaching relationships and poor outcomes. Delivering more than was promised creates an even stronger bond. Going beyond the expected minimum is a great way to build rapport and trust. For example, coaches may contact clients by e-mail between coaching sessions to congratulate them or to remind them of something important. Offering the opportunity for an occasional extra coaching session or check-in at no extra charge is a real "wow!"

and a great relationship builder. When clients e-mail or contact a coach, it is best practice to respond within 24 hours business hours, if only to acknowledge the contact and to promise a date and time for a more thoughtful response.

## The Client Finds the Answers, as Far as Is Possible

The more that clients, in creative collaboration with their coaches, discover new insights, perspectives, strengths, goals, and plans, and the more they design their own strategies for growth and change, the more autonomous and competent they become.

When clients need to gain knowledge or learn new skills to move forward, it's important to preserve client autonomy when helping them gain knowledge and skills. If coaches have relevant knowledge and expertise, they ask permission to offer their expertise and teaching, while leaving clients in control of their decision and choices. If coaches do not have relevant expertise and knowledge, coaches can help clients find and pursue appropriate knowledge and expertise from other sources.

Coaching is about fostering growth, not forcing it. It can be especially difficult to encourage clients to find their own answers when the coach has expertise in particular areas (e.g., diabetes, weight loss). Clients may ask for advice in managing medical conditions, making medical decisions, or learning new skills (e.g., strength training or meditation). The more expertise one has, the easier it is to slip into the role of expert or advisor and to insist on what clients must work on or do. Given that telling clients what to do can damage trust, create resistance, and hold back self-determination, imagine that the client is sitting in the driver's seat, and the coach is offering expert information to consider from the passenger seat, rather than grabbing the steering wheel and deciding what a client should do or where a client should go next

There is a growing and hopeful shift in the healthcare industry to become more client-centered (patient-centered) and allow for increased client determination and self-discovery. In a systematic review on health and wellness coaching, 61% of coaching processes could be described as patient-centered, 45% allow clients to determine their own goals, and 42% encourage self-discovery (Wolever et al., 2013). The healthcare field still has a long way to shift away from top-down and authoritative directing, prescribing, and educating in order to foster autonomy, competence, and self-determination.

When it is given, information should be offered in response to a request or offered as a choice, and it should almost always be framed as a possibility rather than as a prescription. Allowing the client to make the choice supports autonomy and is mutually constructive for coaches and clients alike. Something is wrong in the relationship when coaches are working harder or talking more than their clients in coaching sessions, whether to create goals, figure out strategies, or develop the case for change.

## COACHING CASE

Coach Carl notices that his client, Wendy Well, seems frantic at the beginning of their coaching session. When he mentions this, she acknowledges that it has been a hectic day and she is feeling stressed. Carl has taught many stress management courses in workplace wellness programs and could easily make suggestions about stress reduction techniques that Wendy could use. Instead, Carl uses the coach approach and asks Wendy what she could like to do in this situation and what would be most helpful as his support. Wendy, still frenzied, responds saying she's not really certain; stress just seems to be a way of life. Next, balancing the expert approach with the coach approach, Carl asks Wendy whether she would like to discuss some quick techniques to tame her frenzy right now. Wendy agrees. Carl remembers the importance of allowing a client to feel autonomous and says the following: "One thing that has been helpful to my clients in the past is to pause for 60 seconds to do some deep breathing. Another client really enjoyed taking a moment to explore what she was grateful for. And another got a real boost from doing a simple chair yoga exercise. Which of these appeals to you? Did any give you an idea for something you could do right now that would work for you?"

## Confidentiality Is Crucial

The coaching relationship is built on a foundation of confidentiality. Clients need to know that the information they share with their coaches will not be shared with others. A coach should make this clear both orally and in writing. Some clients may initially be intimidated or uncomfortable about personal disclosure. It is up to the coach to create a safe place by establishing a policy of confidentiality from the beginning.

There may be instances when a client wants to share something personal but does not want it to be recorded in your paper, electronic, or web client files. A client may say something like, "I want to tell you something, but I don't want it to be written down or be part of my record." It is important to exclude such confidences from records or coaching notes but only if it does not create liability (i.e., it is a health-endangering or illegal behavior).

Additionally, the Health Insurance Portability and Accountability Act of 1996 (HIPAA) requires that individuals, organizations, and agencies that meet the definition of a covered entity under HIPAA must comply with the law's requirements to protect the privacy and security of health information and must respect certain rights with respect to individuals' health information. This includes providers such as doctors, clinics, psychologists, dentists, chiropractors, nursing homes, and pharmacies if they transmit any information in an electronic form in connection with a transaction for which the federal government's U.S. Department of Health and Human Services has adopted a standard. It would be wise for any coach engaging in health and wellness-related coaching to be aware of the requirements of HIPAA. Learn more at www.hhs.gov.

## Be Authentic

Authenticity is not only the best policy, it is the *only* policy when it comes to coaching. Clients and coaches alike should agree to "share what is there" with courage, because honest communication leads to learning and growth. However, coaches should never be or sound critical or judgmental. Coaches are called to share thoughts, feelings, and intuitions with compassion, empathy, and care. A trusting and meaningful coaching relationship is built through authentic inquiries and reflections.

## Mindfulness

Mindfulness is the nonjudgmental awareness of what is happening in the present moment. The topic of mindfulness is now supported by a large body of knowledge and practice; it is considered a health-promoting intervention that enhances the coaching process. In order to increase client awareness of the critical variables which influence their success, coaches ask questions, give feedback, and co-create assignments that increase client mindfulness.

More often than not, clients are not fully aware of and awake to *where they are and what they are doing*. That's because people often walk around on automatic pilot. When they are eating, they may simultaneously be reading, working, or worrying about past or future events instead of tasting fully each bite of food. When they are working out, they may be thinking about all they have to do that day instead of being in tune with their bodies and what they are doing.

Mindfulness is a way to break free from being on autopilot. By paying attention to our thoughts, feelings, behaviors, relationships, and environments without judgment or condemnation, we wake up to the experience of what's going on around us and within us *while it's actually happening*. This frees us to make informed decisions about new directions.

Everyone has the ability to be mindful. For example, eating provides a wonderful opportunity to become mindful. Instead of rushing through meals or snacks, doing two things at once with hardly a thought as to what we are eating, where the food comes from, or how it will impact our bodies, minds, and spirits, we can slow down and pay attention in ways that increase enjoyment, change our relationship to food, and make us more conscious of our consumption. Such mindfulness can lead not only to improved eating habits but also to fuller experiences in other areas of life. Increased mindfulness in one area leads to increased mindfulness in all areas.

One strategy for promoting mindfulness is to ensure that a coach's working space has minimal distractions, (e.g., foot traffic, noise, phone, and computer alerts) that could interfere with one's ability to remain present and focused. Relaxation and reminder techniques can assist you in leaving your thoughts and concerns "at the door" in order to focus entirely on the client. "Set your intention to pay attention" is a great refrain to use prior to each coaching session.

To give clients an experience of mindfulness during coaching sessions, coaches may want to include mindfulness exercises. For example, coaches may want to start their coaching conversations with a minute of silence and breath work. They may also choose to guide clients to discover an object with a beginner's mind. For example, the coach can guide clients to experience a raisin very slowly by examining its surface, feeling its texture, smelling it, etc. Clients can then be told to put it in their mouths and get a sense of it on their tongues. Then and only then should they take the first bite, eating it as slowly as possible, noticing each sensation as it comes. This exercise allows clients to awaken from their automatic reactions to food which may not support healthy eating.

By increasing mindfulness during coaching sessions, clients learn to increase mindfulness in their daily experiences. They naturally grow to pay more attention not only to the food but also to the many dynamics of health, wellness, and life. Jon Kabat-Zinn (2005) writes:

"When, through the practice of mindfulness, we learn to listen to the body through all its sense doors, as well as to attend to the flow of our thoughts and feelings, we are beginning the process of reestablishing and strengthening connectedness within our own inner landscape. That attention nurtures a familiarity and an intimacy with our lives unfolding at the level of what we call body and what we call mind that depends and strengthens well-being and a sense of ease in our relationship to whatever is unfolding in our lives from moment to moment. We thus move from dis-ease, including outright disease, to greater ease and harmony and, as we shall see, greater health." (p. 123)

Because it is important to be mindful in the everyday moments of our lives, coaches may want to offer advice to clients on how they can elevate mindfulness between coaching sessions. For example, clients can ask themselves the following questions before, during, and after eating:

- Where am I?
- What is my body position?
- What is going on around me?
- Am I really hungry?
- What does the food look, smell, feel, and taste like?
- What am I thinking about?
- What am I feeling?
- What do I really want to eat?
- How can I enhance my experience of eating?

Coaches cannot facilitate the development of mindfulness in their clients unless they become mindful. It is only in the practice of mindfulness that we can come to understand the process and its effect on health, fitness, and wellness. By practicing mindfulness in our everyday lives and showing up mindfully with clients, coaches enable clients to learn, grow, and develop beyond what they might otherwise have imagined possible.

Mindfulness is also a critical ingredient for coaches in managing their emotions during coaching sessions. The more a coach knows about what is going on with themselves, the less they will allow their own events, feelings, opinions, and worries to get in the way of being present in the moment.

When clients trigger an emotional response, a coach needs to notice those feelings and then gently set them aside, staying focused on the client. Examining those feelings later outside the coaching session—alone or with a mentor coach—is important to a coach's development.

Here are some tips for activating mindfulness before coaching sessions:

- Take three deep breaths.
- Close eyes for five seconds.
- Become aware of your breathing.
- Say to yourself:
  - I am grateful for this opportunity to connect and make a difference.

- I have an opportunity to make a pivotal contribution.
- I am open to and curious about what will unfold.

## Three Core Coaching Skills

Although different coaching models and platforms have their own inventory, language, and description of what's in the coaching repertoire, three coaching skills are consistently found across platforms, and these form the basis for developing the coaching relationship. They are introduced here and are explored again from different angles in later chapters.

## Mindful Listening

Mindful listening is perhaps the most important of all coaching skills. It is certainly a critical component in building trust and rapport with a client. Additionally, it is the most important element in improving the quality of the conversation between coach and client. When coaches are distracted, whether physically, intellectually, emotionally, or spiritually, the coaching relationship suffers.

Listening that brings full, nonjudgmental awareness of what someone is saying in the present moment is the hallmark of great coaching. Indeed, there may be no other relationship in our clients' lives where they are heard in the way they are heard by coaches. People seldom have the undivided, nonjudgmental attention of anyone, even for brief periods of time. Trying to do two things at once may cause us to lose strands of the conversation and degrade the quality of our inquiries and reflections. And clients can tell when coaches are not 100% present. If coaches fail to pay full attention, their energy becomes less focused and engaging. Clients will often accept this low level of focus and engagement because it is the norm in modern culture. It's up to the coach to take the conversation to a higher level by paying full attention.

Paying attention is about more than just listening to or looking at the client. In the overstimulated environment of today, brains have become "wired into a state of frenzy and chronic distraction"

(Hammerness & Moore, 2012). Coaches and clients need to retrain their brains to sustain attention to be truly mindful in the present moment. Mindfulness is the nonjudgmental awareness of what is happening in the present moment. Mindfulness is a way to break free from being on autopilot or from being frenzied and caught up in the core emotions of anxiety, sadness, and anger. By paying attention to one's thoughts, feelings, behaviors, relationships, and environments without judgment or condemnation, it is possible to wake up to the experience of what's going on around us and within us while it's actually happening. This frees one to make informed decisions about new directions. Therefore, mindfulness is important for both the coach and client in the coaching session.

Mindful listening involves listening for the meaningful whole, including such diverse elements as a client's best experiences, core values, significant moments, feelings, current challenges, and future dreams. In addition, the stories clients tell enable coaches to tap into their intuition in order to generate better questions and more evocative reflections. These are the raw materials of coaching. Masterful coaches listen to the words and to the truth beyond the words. It is important to not only listen to the facts (cognitive listening) but also to the feelings and needs behind the facts (affective listening). "The facts, ma'am, just the facts," may be suitable for detective work, but it is never enough for coaching. Clients' moods, emotions, tones, energy, body language, hesitations, and pacing provide important clues. Listening for trends and repeated patterns can lead to important insights.

Here are some quick tips for mindful listening:

- Do not think about what you will say next until your client has spoken the last word of his or her thought.
- Pause after your client has spoken.
- Weave the client's last words into the next step.
- Weave the client's story into later steps.
- Listen for emotions as well as facts.
- Do not interrupt (except in the rare moment when your client wanders off track).
- Mirror what the client has said to confirm your understanding.

Mindfulness is also a critical skill for coaches in managing their emotions during coaching sessions. The more coaches are aware of their inner experience, the less they will allow their own experiences, feelings, opinions, and worries to get in the way of being present in the moment. When clients trigger an emotional response for the coach, a mindful coach will notice those feelings and gently set them aside to stay focused wholly on the client. Following the coaching session, the coach can then examine those feelings alone or with a mentor coach. Coaches must silence the voices in their own heads so they can actively pay attention to the voice of the client. "Listen until I don't exist" is the motto of great coaches. That's because they set aside their agendas in order to pay singular attention to their clients' agendas. Coaches describe the experience as both liberating and deep. Mindful listening is transformational, not only for the client but also for the coach.

## COACHING CASE

Coach Carl has had a busy day of coaching; clients were scheduled for him back to back with barely a moment's break in between. As if that weren't enough to make him feel frenzied, Carl just finished a session with his most difficult client and is beginning to regret one of the questions he asked his client because it seemed to take the session off track. However, Carl has another coaching session with Wendy Well in two minutes and knows that he needs to be mindful and calm for her. He takes three slow, deep breaths, being mindful of each breath in and out. Next, he focuses on a mantra: "I am grateful for this opportunity to connect and make a difference. I am open and curious about what will unfold. I choose to be present."

By increasing mindfulness during coaching sessions, clients learn to increase mindfulness in their daily experiences. They naturally grow to pay more attention not only to eating and exercising but

also to the many dynamics of health, wellness, and life. Thich Nhat Hanh (1999) writes:

> Feelings, whether of compassion or irritation, should be welcomed, recognized, and treated on an absolutely equal basis; because both are ourselves. The tangerine I am eating is me. The mustard greens I am planting are me. I plant with all my heart and mind. I clean this teapot with the kind of attention I would have were I giving the baby Buddha or Jesus a bath. Nothing should be treated more carefully than anything else. In mindfulness, compassion, irritation, mustard green plant, and teapot are all sacred."

> –Thich Nhat Hanh, The Miracle of Mindfulness: An Introduction to the Practice of Meditation

## Open-Ended Inquiry

To enable clients to open up and explore their stories, it's important to ask open-ended questions. Open-ended questions elicit long, narrative answers. Closed-ended questions elicit short, "sound-bite" answers.

## COACHING CASE

### Closed-Ended Questions

Coach Carl is checking in with Wendy Well to see how she did with her goals from last week. "Did you eat salad for lunch last week?" he asks.

"Yes," she replies.

"OK, great!" says Carl, "Did you enjoy it?"

"Yes" she replies again.

"Good. Will you do it again next week?" he asks.

"Probably not," she says.

Closed-ended questions can lead to a dead-end, lifeless conversation, creating more work for the coach and fewer insights for the client.

"What" and "how" are often the best ways to begin open-ended questions because they encourage storytelling. Because stories are the stuff that move people to change, "what" and "how" are the starting points for great coaching questions. "Why" questions are often not as useful, as they tend to provoke analysis rather than storytelling. They may also evoke resistance because they can suggest judgment. For example, asking "Why did you eat the whole cake?" may cause a client to respond defensively. "Why" questions, however, can be powerful when deployed to elicit autonomous motivation. You can connect clients to their deepest motivators by asking, "Why do you treasure your vision and goals, and why do they matter deeply?"

Although coaches use more open than closed questions, there is a place for closed questions. For example, when coaches ask clients whether they want to commit, whether it is to a vision, strategy, or goal—"Are you ready to move forward?"

Do not rush clients through the telling of their stories sparked by open-ended inquiry. By taking the time to evoke and listen to a client's stories, a coach reflects a genuine interest in a client's experience and aspirations. It's never helpful to grill a client with a series of questions, especially one right after another. Instead of asking clients to cut to the chase, invite clients to elaborate in order to tease out the nuances, meanings, and treasures in their stories. Displaying curiosity is a wonderful way to help a client open up. It's also not helpful to make assumptions or launch too quickly into advice giving. Take the time to listen to what's being said, to what's not being said, and to what clients may want to say, gently guiding them to discover their own answers. Great inquiries elicit what is on the client's mind rather than what is on the coach's mind.

When clients avoid or fail to respond to a question, or if you think they aren't being totally authentic in their answer, drop it and come back to it at another time. If this happens consistently regarding the same issue, you may want to share this perception with your client without judgment. Accept the client's decision about what to share and what to keep private.

## Examples of Open-Ended Inquiry

- What would you like your wellness to look like in three months, one year, two years, five years, etc.?
- What are the top three values in your life?
- What are the top three goals in your life?
- What part of your life is most important to you?
- What would you like less of in your life?
- What would you like more of in your life?
- What excites you?
- What would you like to accomplish in the next three months?
- What motivators are important enough to you to enable you to overcome your obstacles meet your goals?
- What would your life be like if you achieve these goals?
- What would your life be like if you do not achieve these goals?
- What is the best case scenario?
- What is the worst case scenario?
- What will it take for you to make changes?
- What have you tried and succeeded to accomplish in your life that is similar to this goal?
- What are some new possibilities that you haven't considered before?
- What do you think is the best possible outcome of our coaching program?
- What do you think is the likely outcome of our coaching program?
- What do you think is the worst possible outcome of our coaching program?
- What would you like the outcome of our coaching program to be?
- What is happening when you feel _____?
- What are the triggers that are stimulating you to feel _____?
- What would it take to deal with your feelings of _____?
- What is holding you back or standing in your way? How is it holding you back?
- What are you afraid of?
- What is at risk for you?
- What is more important to you than meeting this goal?

- What would make this the right time for you to do this?
- What is on your plate right now that may be getting in the way, this week, this next month, in the next three months, etc.?
- What would you like to do?
- What are you able to do to overcome _____ or meet your goal?
- What are you willing to do to overcome _____ or meet your goal?
- What do you want to do to overcome _____ or meet your goal?
- What can I do to best help you today (or in our coaching program)?
- What might I do better to help you today (or in our coaching program)?
- What would your life be like if you do not achieve this goal?
- What would your life be like if you do achieve this goal?
- What is the best case scenario if you achieve this goal?
- What is the worst case scenario if you don't achieve this goal?
- What might be wrong about this goal?
- What might be right about this goal?
- What will it take for you to reach this goal?
- What would it take for you to be ready to change?
- What motivator is important enough to you to help you reach this goal?
- What can you/we learn from this?
- What is the solution here?
- In the next week, what could you think about or do that would move you forward?
- What have you tried and succeeded to accomplish in your life that is similar to this goal?
- What are some new possibilities that you haven't considered before?

## Perceptive Reflections

Asking too many questions of any sort in a row can lead to a client feeling interrogated. Perceptive reflections are another form of listening. They enable clients to hear what they are saying from the vantage point of another person. This process is often

**COACHING CASE**

**Open-Ended Inquiry**

Coach Carl is checking in with Wendy Well to see what she learned from her goals over the last week. "Tell me about what happened with your goal of eating lunch salads last week. What went well?" he inquires.

"I had salad for lunch every day last week. I experimented with putting new sources of protein on it every day and even tried not having any salad dressing," she replies.

"Sounds as though the experimenting went well," says Carl. "What did you enjoy about that?"

"I was really surprised that with the right combination of things, the salad was just as fulfilling as the hamburger or pizza I would usually get," she answered.

"Good. What will you do with this learning next week?" he asks.

"I would like to have salad for lunch Monday through Thursday next week. But Friday is my coworker's birthday and I know that we'll have pizza that day to celebrate. Still, I think I'll experiment with veggies instead of pepperoni on the pizza," she says.

more provocative and transformational than inquiry because it causes clients to connect more deeply to their emotions and the truth of the matter.

When coaches ask questions, clients objectively think about and formulate an answer before responding. The "CEO" (or analytical) region of the brain (mostly the left prefrontal cortex) is activated as people are drawn into their analytical minds.

When coaches perceptively paraphrase and reflect what they think clients are saying, clients react with a deeper, more emotional response generated from the limbic region of the brain where emotions, rewards, and pleasure are regulated. The combination of questions and reflections may integrate the use of higher and lower brain regions.

The purpose of perceptive reflections is to elicit ideas and conversation in the client which support change. Instead of the coach making the case for change, the client is encouraged to pick up the ball and run with it. When the case for change comes from the client rather than the coach, rapid progress can be made in the direction of desired outcomes.

It's not important to focus on making reflections that are "right" or "perfect." If the reflection is accurate, clients agree. If it is off target, clients disagree. Either way, the reflection moves clients forward and engages them in the search for more self-awareness, higher well-being, and the "best me."

The simplest reflection is to restate what a client says in more or less his or her own words. Like a mirror, such simple reflections enable clients to see themselves more clearly and make adjustments if they so desire. Other, more complex reflections are intentionally designed to be more evocative. They communicate not only that the coach is actively listening but also that the coach is noticing things the client may be overlooking. They can serve to make the prospect of change sound bigger, brighter, or more inviting. They enable clients to stop and consider whether they want to spend more time on those issues.

### Examples of Simple Perceptive Reflections

Wendy Well: "I am worried about setting a running goal because I haven't run since high school."

Coach Carl: "You are concerned about running because it has been a long time since you last ran."

Wendy Well: "I'm looking forward to setting a running goal because I haven't run since high school but I used enjoy it a lot."

Coach Carl: "You remember enjoying running in high school, and look forward to feeling that way again."

Wendy Well: "I'm so glad I set that running goal. I haven't felt this good since high school."

Coach Carl: "You are happy that you set goal because running makes you feel good."

In the chapter, "Harnessing Motivation to Build Self-Efficacy," we describe additional forms of perceptive reflections: empathy, amplified, double-sided, and shifted-focus.

## Additional Relationship-Building Tools

Along with mindful listening, open-ended inquires, and perceptive reflections are high-impact coaching tools, here are several more tools for enhancing client progress.

### Positive Reframing

Positive reframing means framing a client's experiences in positive terms. Once the conversation takes a positive turn, it is easier to engage in brainstorming, action planning, and forward movement. It is a natural human tendency to look at, focus on, and talk about problems. Indeed, many people who come to coaching would say they want help with a problem. "I'm overweight," "I'm out of shape," and "I'm stressed out" are three of the most common complaints in the health and wellness arena.

From week to week, many clients also want to start the coaching conversation with a problem as the issue of the day. For example, "I blew my diet," "I didn't exercise like I said I would," and "I took no time for myself this week." Masterful coaches avoid the temptation to respond to such complaints with a root-cause problem analysis, which can be demoralizing, overwhelming, and counterproductive.

Instead of inspiring and empowering change, problem analysis can weigh people down with more reasons not to change. Without dismissing people's problems, masterful coaches know how to reframe the conversation in positive terms.

At times, clients need to be reminded that setbacks are an essential part of the change process. When learning to walk, infants fall many times. These are not failures, but essential lessons that help them learn how to walk. By encouraging clients to positively reframe, a coach can enable them not only to get back on track but also to avoid

## COACHING CASE

As she shares her experience in working on her goals last week, Wendy Well is frustrated and disappointed.

"I was certain that I would be able to eat salad for lunch most days last week. I'd had such a good experience with it last week, and this week I blew it! I'm so mad at myself!"

"I hear that you are disappointed and frustrated because you really wanted to feel successful with this goal," Carl responds. "Tell me about the good choices you did make last week."

"Well, I did choose to have vegetables on the pizza we had during the celebration on Friday," she reflects.

"And what good came from that?" Carl asks curiously.

"You know, I really enjoyed the banana peppers; I didn't even miss the pepperoni," she recalls with a smile.

becoming attached to feelings of failure, even if they think they failed.

## Silence

One thing is certain—if the coach is talking, the coach is not listening. Given the importance of listening in coaching, it's vital that coaches become comfortable with silence. When clients are speaking, do not interrupt them and/or think about what to say next. After asking a question, do not talk again before the client answers. Be prepared for the surprises of silence! It is a wonderful gift and a core tool in coaching. In masterful coaching sessions, clients talk more than twice as much as coaches. Nicola Stevens (2005) encourages coaches to remember the acronym, "WAIT—Why am I talking?" (p. 161).

Silence evokes deeper exploration by sending the empowering message without words, "I believe

that you can figure this out by going deeper." Often, silence will lead to new insights and directional shifts that clients and coaches may have never anticipated. Silence supports the client in providing a sense of autonomy and sends the message the coach is confident in the client's competence.

## Humor and Playfulness

Although coaching is serious business with serious goals in which people are seriously invested, this does not mean the coaching conversation itself needs to have a serious tone. In fact, a consistently serious tone may cause clients to dread their coaching sessions and consequently fail to connect and progress.

The more often a coach can make clients laugh and see the lighter side of their challenges and opportunities, the more they will open themselves up to change. A playful approach can make clients more open to experimentation and to trial and correction. Be careful not to joke about something that may make a client feel vulnerable. Use empathy to distinguish between those areas that are ripe for humor and those that may make your client feel worse if treated too lightly. Be sure clients never think you're laughing at them. It's fair game, though, to laugh at yourself!

## Championing

At all times coaches champion their clients' ability to realize their goals, especially when they lack self-efficacy. When the coach has an upbeat and energetic attitude, combined with a positive outlook, clients are more able to find the courage for change. Coaching is a hope-inspiring relationship. Dave Buck (2004), President of CoachVille, describes this dynamic as follows: "The coach's certainty is greater than the client's doubt." That dynamic is what attracts clients to masterful coaches. When clients are struggling, coaches reassure them that different people move toward mastery of health, fitness, or wellness at different speeds and at different times in their lives. When they are ready, they can and will succeed. As the coach, work to facilitate a client's movement at a time and speed that is comfortable yet challenging. This is the "flow zone" that will enable clients to achieve the goals they have set for themselves.

## COACHING CASE

Coach Carl champions Wendy Well:

- At the beginning of the coaching session: "I've looked forward to speaking with you today Wendy. You are so engaged in our work together, and I'm always eager to see what insights you have."
- During the coaching session: "How exciting to hear that you were willing to continue with your vegetable experiment. You are tenacious!"
- At the close of the coaching session: "Today your strengths of curiosity and compassion for yourself were definitely present."

Continually focus on and champion the positive changes, without dwelling too long on the negatives. Coaching is about possibilities, action, and learning, not blame and shame.

## Solicit Input and Suggestions

It is important to ask clients to share input and make suggestions on how the coaching process can be made more productive and enjoyable. Soliciting input builds the coaching relationship by making it clear to a client that the coach is totally devoted to the client's success. Frequently ask, "What was most valuable about today's session?" and "How could our sessions work better for you?" Listen for what is unspoken but conveyed in a client's tone and hesitations. Ask for clarification if it seems there might be an issue or shift in energy. Keep private notes and follow-up on the points raised as soon as possible.

Most new coaches experience clients who go missing in action, not showing up for coaching sessions or disappearing without explanation. By asking clients at the outset of the coaching program

to make you the first to know if anything isn't working; then there is an opening to talk about their concerns rather than act them out by not showing up. Upon the receipt of criticism, listen for and respond to needs that are going unmet for the client. Thank clients for their input and use it to get better as a coach. Consult a mentor or engage in coaching supervision to develop strategies to improve. Never jump to conclusions; always ask for the client's perceptions, interpretations, and points of view.

## COACHING CASE

Wendy Well has been doing so well on her eating goals that Coach Carl decides he won't ask about how she did this week. He fears that she'll get bored with the coaching relationship if they keep talking about the same thing each week or, worse yet, will seem like a nag. Wendy came to the coaching session today eager to talk about her eating goals because she'd had a huge breakthrough in her understanding of what was driving her to snack in the afternoons. She was disappointed that Carl didn't even ask about those goals today because she doesn't have anyone else in her life with whom she can explore these kinds of topics. "I hope Carl isn't getting bored with me since I've been working on the same eating goal for several weeks," she worries.

## References

Baumeister, R., & Leary, M. R. (1995). The need to belong: Desire for interpersonal attachments as a fundamental human motivation, *Psychological Bulletin, 117*(3), 497–529.

Buck, D. (2004). The language of coaching. In *So just what is coaching, anyway?* Retrieved October 16, 2008 from http://www.lazarconsulting.com/resources .interview.042805.html

De Haan, E. (2008). *Relational coaching.* West Sussex, England: John Wiley & Sons.

Dotlich, D., & Cairo, P. (1999). *Action coaching: How to leverage individual performance for company success.* San Francisco: Jossey-Bass.

Empathy. (n.d.). In *Merriam Webster's online dictionary* (11th ed.). Retrieved April 1, 2014 from http://www.merriam-webster.com/dictionary/empathy

Gallwey, W. T. (2000). *The inner game of work.* New York: Random House.

Hammerness, P., & Moore, M. (2012). *Organize your mind, organize your life.* New York: Harlequin.

International Association of Coaching. (2014). *Coaching masteries.* Retrieved March 25, 2014 from http://www.certifiedcoach.org/index.php/get_certified/the_iac_coaching_masteries_overview/

International Coach Federation. (2014). *Coaching competencies.* Retrieved March 25, 2014 from http://coachfederation.org/credential/landing.cfm?ItemNumber=2206&navItemNumber=576

Kabat-Zinn, J. (2005). *Coming to our senses: Healing ourselves and the world through mindfulness.* New York: Hyperion.

Norcross, J., & Lambert, M. (2010). Evidence-based therapy relationships. In J. Norcross (Ed.), *Evidence-based therapy relationships* (pp. 1–4). Rockville, MD: Substance Abuse and Mental Health Services Administration.

Perry, J. (2005). *The fan club game: Tap your most powerful resource; enjoy a full-filling practice.* Laguna Hills, CA: CreativeU Publishing.

Pity. (n.d.). In *Merriam Webster's online dictionary.* Retrieved April 1, 2014 from http://www.merriam-webster.com/dictionary/pity

Rogers, C. R. (1995). *On becoming a person: A therapist's view of psychotherapy.* New York: Houghton Mifflin.

Ryan, R., Patrick, H., Deci, E., & Williams, G. (2008). Facilitating health behaviour change and its maintenance: Interventions based on self-determination theory. *The European Health Psychologist, 10,* 2–5.

Silsbee, D. (2008). *Presence-based coaching.* San Francisco: Jossey-Bass.

Stevens, N. (2005). *Learn to coach: The skills you need to coach for personal and professional development.* Oxford, United Kingdom: How To Books.

Sympathy. (n.d.). In *Merriam Webster's online dictionary* (11th ed.). Retrieved April 1, 2014 from http://www.merriam-webster.com/dictionary/sympathy

Tschannen-Moran, M. (2004). *Trust matters: Leadership for successful schools.* San Francisco: Jossey-Bass.

U.S. Department of Health and Human Services. (n.d.). *Health information privacy.* Retrieved April 1, 2014 from http://www.hhs.gov/ocr/privacy/hipaa/understanding/coveredentities/index.html

Wolever, R., Simmons, L., Sforzo, G., Dill, D., Kaye, M., Bechard, E., … Yang, N. (2013). A systematic review of the literature on health and wellness coaching: Defining a key behavioral intervention in healthcare. *Global Advances in Health and Medicine, 2*(4), 38–57.

Zeus, P., & Skiffington, S. (2000). *The complete guide to coaching at work.* New York: McGraw-Hill.

# CHAPTER 3

# Coaching Presence

*"Presence is more than just being there."*

— MALCOLM FORBES

## Defining Coaching Presence

Tim Gallwey (2000) defines coaching as "the art of creating an environment, through conversation and a way of being, that facilitates the process by which a person can move toward desired goals in a fulfilling manner." Gallwey goes on to note that this "requires one essential ingredient that cannot be taught: caring not only for external results but for the person being coached" (p. 177).

This definition highlights that coaching supports client growth and change not only by what coaches do (have conversations with clients) but also by who coaches are (a way of being with people). It is concerned not only with results but also with the person seeking to achieve those results. The two always go hand in hand. Coaching presence, therefore, is a way of being with clients (mindful, empathetic, warm, calm, zestful, fun, and courageous) that facilitates growth and change through connection. Failure to have a full coaching presence with clients undermines the impact of coaching sessions. If a client partnership is not successful, it may have less to do with techniques than with the nature of a coach's presence.

The International Coach Federation also recognizes coaching presence as a core coaching competency, the "ability to be fully conscious and create spontaneous relationship with the client, employing a style that is open, flexible and confident." To this end, the ICF indicates that a professional coach:

- Is present and flexible during the coaching process, dancing in the moment
- Accesses one's intuition and trusts one's inner knowing—"goes with the gut"
- Is open to not knowing and takes risks
- Sees many ways to work with the client and chooses in the moment what is most effective

- Uses humor effectively to create lightness and energy
- Confidently shifts perspectives and experiments with new possibilities for own action
- Demonstrates confidence in working with strong emotions and can self-manage and not be overpowered by or enmeshed in clients' emotions

That's why it's so important for coaches to develop their own empowering frameworks or philosophical principles in their work with clients. Thomas Leonard (2002), a founder of the modern life coaching movement, is famous for suggesting the following notions:

1. It's all solvable or it's not.
2. Risk is always reducible.
3. There's usually a better way.
4. Success is a byproduct.
5. Emotions are our teachers.
6. Inklings are higher intelligence.
7. The answer is somewhere.
8. Self-confidence can be arranged.
9. Problems are immediate opportunities.
10. People are doing their very best, even when they seem not to be.

Frameworks on which coaches lean empower clients in movement, growth, and connection. They undergird what is described as the "quality of presence" that leads to "growth-fostering" or "growth-enhancing" relationships (Jordan, Walker, & Hartling, 2004). Clients learn and grow not only because of what coaches do but also because of who coaches are being.

## Being Skills

Coaching presence is developed through practice of using relational qualities called "being skills." They are the skills coaches use to build growth-promoting relationships and also represent a coach's way of being when at his or her most authentic.

When coaches cultivate a strong coaching presence, grounded in being skills, they possess a

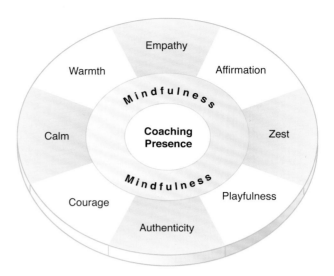

**Figure 3.1.** Illustrates how the "being" skills of coaching presence relate to one another. Surrounding the core of coaching presence is mindfulness, which determines how the coach shows up for coaching and how the other skills are engaged. Around the perimeter, the being skills are arranged in ways that show the connections as well as the distinctions between them.

calm, confident energy that is radiated outward to clients. "Don't just do something, stand there!" is a Buddhist saying that expresses this understanding. By modeling the being skills and the coach's trust in the client's ability to succeed, the coach shifts from coaching competence to coaching mastery. The energy of mastery infuses clients with the self-efficacy clients need to move forward successfully with their vision and goals.

These being skills include such critical qualities as mindfulness, empathy, warmth, affirmation, calm, zest, playfulness, courage, and authenticity. We describe these qualities of being as "skills" because they are qualities that can be chosen, valued, and strengthened in the course of a coach's professional development (Fig. 3.1).

## Mindfulness

Masterful coaching requires mindfulness, or a nonjudgmental awareness of what is happening in the present moment. "When one is mindful, one is actively engaged in the present and sensitive to both context and perspective. The mindful condition is both the result of, and the continuing cause of, actively noticing new things" (Langer & Carson, 2006).

Being fully aware and awake in this way is a prerequisite for everything a coach does. If the coach is not mindful, he or she will not be skillful enough to assist clients in engaging in a deep coach-client relationship that will enable them to reach their vision and goals. It is the task of the coach to pay full attention while suspending judgment and using empathy, inquiry, and reflections. In this way, mindfulness requires two components: self-regulation in order to pay attention in the moment and a posture of curiosity, openness, and acceptance.

A good starting point for developing mindfulness is to begin tuning into the signals sent by our bodies, which work ceaselessly to get our attention. Negative emotions and physical sensations indicate that some of our needs are not being met, whereas positive emotions and physical sensations are signs that they are.

Body intelligence is about having the awareness, knowledge of, and engagement in health habits that generate physical energy and thriving (Gavin & Moore, 2010). To develop both emotional and body intelligence and increase mindfulness, one can move one's conscious attention into a "brainset" that Harvard psychologist Shelley Carson calls the "open awareness" brain state (Fig. 3.2).

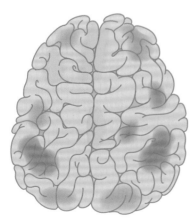

**Figure 3.2.** Note that the prefrontal cortex is blue, signifying that its activity is low. The brain in this state is not thinking, analyzing, or planning; instead, attention moves deep and back into the sensory, or "experiencing," brain regions. Within a coaching conversation, this state of experiencing leads to meaningful and connected engagement with the client. (Source: www.organizeyourmind.com)

Although there is no single strength identified as "mindfulness" by the Values-in-Action (VIA) Signature Strengths Questionnaire, the following strengths, in descending order of correlation, were found by one study to have a significant positive relationship to mindfulness: self-regulation, bravery, integrity, perspective, citizenship, and social intelligence (Silberman, 2007). These correlations suggest intriguing lines of research and development. For example, Silberman discusses ways in which mindfulness may "cultivate a number of strengths simultaneously," perhaps by its ability to quiet "mental chatter."

## Empathy

In the coaching context, empathy is defined as the respectful understanding of another person's experience, including his or her feelings, needs, and desires. It is the core relational dynamic that leads to movement and growth in coaching. An empathetic coach understands and connects with the clients without sharing the experiences, getting hooked, or being hijacked by emotions emerging from within or from the client.

Like mindfulness, empathy allows the coach to suspend all judgment, analysis, suggestions, stories, or motivation to fix things in favor of connecting with and understanding what's alive in and coming up for another human being in the present moment. Someone who is empathetic is:

- Curious without being demanding
- Interested without being intrusive
- Compassionate without being condescending
- Persistent without being impatient

Empathy seeks solely to understand and value another person's experience with respect and compassion. It is the intention to "get with" where another is coming from and nothing else (Jordan et al., 2004). When a client realizes that his or her feelings and needs matter and that he or she is being heard and taken seriously by the coach, a zone of new possibilities is created. It takes work to nurture and maintain this intention. In the interest of being helpful, coaches are especially prone to advise, educate, console, reassure, explain, correct, and solve problems. Although

## COACHING CASE

*In which scenario do you think Wendy received empathy?*

**Scenario 1**

**Wendy Well:** "I am so angry! My boss told me that I have to work a 10-hour shift this week, which means that I can't do my evening walk, and there is no way that I'll be able to eat healthy."

**Expert Carl:** "Well surely there is a way that you can stick to your goals. Don't give up now; you've worked so hard and had such success! You can't have the all-or-nothing attitude. What about walking in the morning instead?"

**Scenario 2**

**Wendy Well:** "I am so angry! My boss told me that I have to work a 10-hour shift this week, which means that I can't do my evening walk and there is no way that I'll be able to eat healthy."

**Coach Carl:** "You are angry and disappointed because you've been so proud of yourself for being consistent with your exercise and eating plans. You are frustrated because you are having a difficult time thinking of strategies maintaining this when your schedule changes. What else are you feeling?"

such behaviors may at times be appropriate and useful in coaching conversations, they interfere with and do not align with a posture of empathy.

Lastly, empathy is good for the coach and the client. Intentionally cultivating nonjudgmental attention leads to connection, which leads to self-regulation and ultimately to greater order and health (Shapiro, Carlson, Astin, & Freedman, 2006).

## Warmth

There is a reciprocal relationship between warmth and empathy. Without warmth, all attempts at empathy will fail. That's because empathy requires a sincere, heartfelt desire to connect with another human being. Obligatory expressions of empathy will be revealed as inauthentic. Likewise, without empathy, all attempts at warmth will fail. That's because warmth requires an awareness of what others are feeling and needing in the present moment.

Warmth comes from what psychologists call "positive regard." It has the power to open up clients, just as sunshine has the power to open flowers. Too little or too much warmth, however, can distress clients, just as too little or too much sunshine can damage flowers. Warmth has to be tailored appropriately for every situation. The key is to radiate just the right amount of warmth in just the right way, so our clients warm up and the coaching process becomes energized.

Warmth generates full engagement. It is a contagious quality of being that enlivens conversations, relationships, and circumstances.

When the coach and client warm up to each other, their energies elevate, ideas are generated, light bulbs go off, and new possibilities get created. When a coach expresses genuine warmth toward a client, it meets the deeply rooted need for connection in the service of self-determination.

## Affirmation

When a coach gives the gift of affirmation, he or she conveys acceptance and appreciation of a client's thoughts, feelings, and choices. This is not the same as affiliation, which implies alignment and agreement with the client's thoughts, feelings, and choices. Masterful coaches extend unfailing affirmation to both themselves and others because they come from a framework that recognizes perfection in every situation. As a biologist would say, "every cell is doing the best it can with the resources it has at hand."

How can each and every situation be perfect, even when it obviously isn't? Each can be perfect by virtue of the fact that every moment is the only moment that can be happening at any moment. There's no way to arrive at any future moment other than through the present moment. Nor is there any way for the present moment to be any different than it is, given all the past moments. Affirmation and acceptance have to do with combining mindfulness and empathy. If we see every situation as perfectly designed for our own movement and growth, then we can embrace every situation for where it comes from and where it leads us. Living fully in the present moment makes perfection easy to affirm.

That is the posture masterful coaches generally take in life, particularly with their clients. They neither disparage themselves nor others. Instead, they continuously come from the transactional framework of "I'm OK, you're OK" (Harris, 2004). The notion that things are not OK is dissipated by recognizing that all unhealthy thoughts, words, and actions are expressions of unmet needs. By hearing the needs that underlie thoughts, words, and actions, masterful coaches can remain unfailingly affirmative in relationship to both themselves and others.

Such perspectives enable coaches to reframe negative energy and challenging circumstances as positive opportunities for movement and growth. Carol Kauffman, PhD, Assistant Clinical Professor at Harvard Medical School, tells the story of a young Asian woman with an eating disorder who came to a session feeling down. She shared that she had spent $40 on food for lunch, which she had vomited up in an alleyway. (This was not the first time she had done this.) When she lifted up her head, she noticed a homeless person not far away, sitting on the ground. Mortified and totally ashamed, she thought, "My goodness, this person doesn't have $40 to spend on food, and look what I've just done." Upon hearing this, Dr. Kauffman responded, "We all have a dark alleyway. That happens to be yours, but we all have one. We all have things in our lives we're ashamed of. You're not alone, and you're not terrible. You're human."

Instead of allowing her client to wallow in her guilt and shame (her place of "not OK"), Dr. Kauffman positively reframed the incident and affirmed her client. Extending unfailing affirmation, regardless of the situation, is about helping clients respond to life's experiences without catastrophizing. Until we can accept every situation as perfectly designed for our own movement and growth, there is no way to be happy and productive in life.

Taken together, empathy, warmth, and affirmation foster an important quality of being necessary for masterful coaching. It doesn't happen through our dispensing expert advice, teaching, consoling, explaining, or correcting. It happens through presence and connection.

## Calm

The word "calm" comes from Greek and Latin roots that refer to "burning heat" or the "heat of the day." To find a resting place in those contexts is the energy of calm, demonstrated and exercised by masterful coaches. It's an energy that comes from connecting with and trusting the unfolding of life, whether on the most personal or universal of levels.

"My certainty is greater than your doubt," says Dave Buck of CoachVille. This idea represents not only an approach masterful coaches take with clients but also their way of being in the world. Calm energy in the fire is the strength that comes from knowing that it's never too late to make a difference. That's what makes it possible for first responders to handle emergencies effectively. Instead of dissolving in the midst of chaos and distress, they maintain perspective and poise in the moment.

Coaches with calm energy are able to step back and observe emotional frenzy in themselves and in their clients and create some degrees of freedom from automatic triggers. This enables them to avoid automatic responses such as fear and anxiety; instead, they notice the emotion, they are present, and they make a choice about the response (Shapiro et al., 2006).

Masterful coaches do the same in their lives and work. They set aside those inner voices, the negative ones that interfere with feeling at peace with oneself, the world, and work. At the start of every day, before every coaching session, and in many other moments in life, they claim the calm energy to make a difference and perhaps even to generate a breakthrough. They believe in and are confident of who they are and what they do. Through being present and open to the unfolding of things to come, they add meaning, purpose, and value. It isn't necessarily easy but it can be done.

## Zest

This energy is different from the energy of calm. It is by nature optimistic and hopeful. It anticipates the best and as a result often generates the best. This is similar to the energy from childhood, when a child is anticipating a special activity or occasion (such as going to the zoo or getting on an airplane), excited with energy and full of zest.

In their book, *The Art of Possibility,* Roz and Ben Zander (2002) write about the importance of "shining eyes" in determining people's level of engagement. Zest looks and feels like eyes shining and smiles sparkling. In spite of life's obvious challenges, masterful coaches radiate zest in ways that generate conversations for change. It's almost impossible for coaches who are filled with zest not to infuse that energy into coaching sessions.

It may not be possible to radiate zestful energy every minute of every day, but masterful coaches do so more often than not. That is what makes a coaching practice successful! People want to get close to and build on the attractive energy of zest. It is self-reinforcing and upward spiraling. Zest supports resilience and self-efficacy in the service of coaching outcomes.

One simple strategy for elevating zest without a total life makeover is to cultivate gratitude. Noticing, remembering, and celebrating good things that happen are powerful antidotes to the patina of bad things that tends to build up over time. Understanding this, masterful coaches stoke their own attitude of gratitude through daily positive practices that build happiness, balance, and self-esteem.

Just as there is a reciprocal relationship between giving and receiving empathy, there is also one between giving and receiving zest. The more things coaches do to fill up their own lives with zest, the more zest they will have to share with others. This is one area in which self-care clearly and directly translates into coaching effectiveness. It is not possible to masterfully coach in a state of feeling overwhelmed, fatigued, stressed, burnt out, or in despair. Without doing the things that make life worth living, including adequate time for rest and recovery, it is hard, if not impossible, to share zestful energy with others.

## Playfulness

Just as empathy, warmth, and affirmation go together, so do playfulness and zest. They may be distinct energies, but they nevertheless support one another. Indeed, it's impossible to sustain zest without playfulness. Playfulness ignites our energy for and engagement with life.

Just as playfulness underlies zest, humor and curiosity underlie playfulness. Without the ability to laugh, especially in the face of life's ironies, incongruities, and adversities, one would seldom find the energy to play. Young children laugh hundreds of times per day; older adults average about 17 times per day. Masterful coaches and other healthy adults know how to laugh and have fun (Balick & Lee, 2003; Wooten, 1996).

Perhaps that's why laughter clubs, which started in India, have turned into a global movement. These groups, which typically meet in the morning, run through a series of laughter patterns that eventually give way (after an initial warmup) to an epidemic of spontaneous giggles, chuckles, and guffaws. Participants report feeling refreshed, relaxed, revitalized, and rejuvenated by the experience.

Coaching is serious business, but that doesn't make it the business of seriousness. Unless we carry ourselves and show up with a certain lightness of being, clients will dread coaching and fail to move forward as they otherwise might.

## Courage and Authenticity

Perhaps the most challenging way of being for many coaches involves courage and authenticity. The word "courage" may conjure up images of judgment, conflict, and pushiness. But being courageous is not about being mean, cruel, or threatening. It's about naming what is present to wake up client's awareness, create connection, and generate movement.

Masterful coaches who understand the difference between being nice and being authentic are able to boldly express their observations, feelings, needs, and requests in the service of client outcomes. They have a genuine way of stepping up to the plate and making conversations real. In concert with all the other coaching strengths, masterful coaches have a fearless, conversational prowess that shakes things loose and stirs things up without offending, violating, blaming, shaming, or demeaning people.

Approaching clients with courage and authenticity may be difficult and intimidating at first, but by shining a light on what "wants to be said," coaches can move clients forward in dynamic and powerful ways. That's because truth is contagious and resonant. As long as we stay with accurate observations free from evaluations and honestly reflect back what we are experiencing and seeing, we enable our clients to honestly gain new awareness and understanding of who they are and what they are facing. As a result, clients can muster the courage to more fully meet their needs.

Guy Corneae expresses this dynamic in the introduction to *Being Genuine: Stop Being Nice, Start Being Real* by Thomas d'Ansembourg (2007), a communication guide for courageous and authentic conversations:

> *Expressing one's truth while respecting others and respecting oneself . . . that is the journey [this book invites us to take] by suggesting that we plunge straight into the heart of how we enter into dialogue with ourselves and others. In it we learn how to reprogram the way we express ourselves. Once that has been done, there comes the joy of being closer to others and closer to ourselves. There is the joy of being open to others. And at the heart of this process lies the possibility of giving up the familiar, even comfortable, confusions with which we so often content ourselves, instead of gaining access to a universe of choice and freedom.* (p. 1)

Such is the key to courageous and authentic conversations in coaching—and in life in general. Having courage in coaching means sharing what is being noticed, felt, needed, and wanted. It often takes time to make this deeper level of connection, but it's worth it. Respectful and genuine interactions with our clients can provoke the change they seek.

## Conveying Coaching Presence

Coaching presence is conveyed in many ways, including word choice, phrasing, pace, body language, facial expressions, and intonation. A variety of factors combine in different ways for each coach to make coaching effective. Masterful coaches use their voices well, both in face-to-face and telephone coaching. Sometimes they use their voices to build excitement with stimulating energy. At other times, they use their voices to calm things down with soothing energy. Either way, coaching presence is conveyed when voice is used in just the right way at just the right time.

Silence, too, is an important part of coaching presence. It conveys comfort, respect, and spaciousness for client experience. Feelings, needs, and desires can take a while to surface and become clear. When coaches are comfortable with silence, their presence becomes more evocative.

One universal trait of coaching presence is the dance between intention and attention in the present moment. Although coaching presence may appear graceful and even effortless in the hands of a masterful coach, it never happens by accident. It takes clear intention and lots of practice. The more coaching we have under our belts, the stronger our presence will be.

None of this works unless coaches are ready, willing, and able to engage. When coaches are exhausted, their strengths desert them. When coaches are rested, all strengths come into play. Paying attention to the rhythm of work and rest, of energy out and in, is an essential part of self-management for conveying coaching presence.

A key factor to consider is the flow of energy in the field between coaches and clients. When presence is conveyed artfully, coaches and clients lean into each other with full engagement. This leaning in can be seen in the eyes and heard in the voice as one thing leads spontaneously to another. If one or the other is leaning out or pulling away, then something isn't working. It's time for the coach to try a different approach.

## Coaching Presence as a Symphony of Strengths

Coaches bring their own unique presence to coaching relationships and conversations. Because no two coaches are exactly the same, no two coaches come from exactly the same frameworks or use the core coaching skills in exactly the same way. Who a coach is being influences and in many respects, determines how he or she connects, moves with the clients, and intuitively dances, generating new possibilities and forward momentum.

One way to think of presence is as the expression of a unique symphony of talents and character strengths. These are the aptitudes or capacities that coaches most value and use most ably. In multiple studies, research has shown a direct relationship between the engagement of a person's character strengths and his or her effectiveness, as well as happiness, in both life and work. That's as true for coaches as it is for anyone else. The more the coach plays to and comes from his or her own strengths, the more powerful and effective the coaching will be. This is not to say that strengths are the only factors that generate one's coaching presence. However, at an early stage of one's evolution as a coach, feeling overwhelmed by how much there is to learn and practice is common. It is vital for new coaches to discover or reconnect with personal strengths and use them to foster one's presence as a coach.

To fully engage our talents and character strengths, it helps to know what they are. One of the more significant contributions of positive psychology over the past 10 years has been the development of classification schemes for human strengths that are similar in both form and function to the *Diagnostic and Statistical Manual of Mental Disorders,* 5th edition (*DSM-5*). What the *DSM-5* is to mental illness, the emerging models for strengths, talents, and virtues are to mental and emotional wellness. One strengths model is StrengthsFinder, a popular workplace model developed by the Gallup organization (Rath, 2007).

Peterson and Seligman (2004) have developed a different model, identifying 24 character strengths, grouped into six large categories called virtues that consistently emerge across history and culture. The virtues are wisdom, courage, humanity, justice, temperance, and transcendence. A free online survey, known as the VIA Signature Strengths Questionnaire, generates a report that identifies a person's character strengths in rank order (from 1 to 24). The top five strengths are called "signature strengths," which interact with each other and most influence a person's presence in the world.

The following summarizes and organizes the 24 character strengths (Peterson & Seligman, 2004) with the addition of coaching perspectives. All strengths and coaching perspectives are valuable, and there is no "right" combination of signature strengths when it comes to masterful coaching. Coaching strengths and perspectives impact every aspect of presence and practice, including who coaches are, how coaches show up for coaching, who coaches attract as clients, and how coaches facilitate clients' movement and growth.

## Wisdom and Knowledge

Cognitive strengths that entail the acquisition and use of knowledge:

### 1. Creativity (originality, ingenuity):

Thinking of novel and productive ways to do things; includes artistic achievement but is not limited to it

*Coaching Perspective:* "I love to think outside the box with my clients, generating novel and productive—even fun—ways of doing things."

### 2. Curiosity (interest, novelty-seeking, openness to experience):

Taking an interest in all of ongoing experience for its own sake; finding subjects and topics fascinating; exploring and discovering

*Coaching Perspective:* "I love to explore all facets of a situation, especially the best situations have to offer, to broaden and build on client strengths."

### 3. Open-mindedness (judgment, critical thinking):

Thinking things through and examining them from all sides; not jumping to conclusions; being able to change one's mind in light of evidence; weighing all evidence fairly

*Coaching Perspective:* "Instead of jumping to conclusions, I love to think things through, adopt different perspectives with my clients, examining them from all sides with no urgency."

### 4. Love of learning:

Mastering new skills, topics, and bodies of knowledge, whether on one's own or formally; obviously related to strength of curiosity but goes beyond it to describe the tendency to add systematically to what one knows

*Coaching Perspective:* "I love to learn new things and assist my clients in learning new things, building on what we know now to master unknown skills, topics, and bodies of knowledge in the future."

### 5. Perspective (wisdom):

Being able to provide wise counsel to others; having ways of looking at the world that make sense to oneself and to other people

*Coaching Perspective:* "I love to make sense of experience, both for myself and with my clients, in meaningful and purposeful ways."

## Courage

Emotional strengths that involve the exercise of will to accomplish goals in the face of opposition, external or internal:

### 6. Bravery (valor):

Not shrinking from threat, challenge, difficulty, or pain; speaking up for what is right, even if there is opposition; acting on convictions, even if unpopular; includes physical bravery but is not limited to it

*Coaching Perspective:* "I am willing to speak the truth in love, holding my clients feet to the fire even when it may be uncomfortable."

### 7. Persistence (perseverance, industriousness):

Finishing what one starts; persisting in a course of action in spite of obstacles; "getting it out the door"; taking pleasure in completing tasks.

*Coaching Perspective:* "I hang in there with my clients until we get the job done. Nothing is impossible; some things just take a little longer."

### 8. Integrity (authenticity, honesty):

Speaking the truth and more broadly, presenting oneself in a genuine way; being without pretense; taking responsibility for one's feelings and actions.

*Coaching Perspective:* "I seek to be genuine in all my communications with clients, especially when I sense there may be feelings, needs, and desires below the surface that want to be spoken."

### 9. Vitality (zest, enthusiasm, vigor, energy):

Approaching life with excitement and energy; not doing things halfway or halfheartedly; living life as an adventure; feeling alive and activated

*Coaching Perspective:* "I love life, and I do everything, including coaching, with excitement and energy. Life is an adventure that I seek to live and share with full engagement. People find that to be infectious."

## Humanity

Interpersonal strengths that involve caring and supporting others:

### 10. Love:

Valuing close relations with others, in particular those in which sharing and caring are reciprocated; being close to people

*Coaching Perspective:* "I love to feel close to people and be in mutually supportive relationships. Warmth is a signature of my coaching style."

### 11. Kindness (generosity, nurturance, care, compassion, altruistic love, "niceness"):

Doing favors and good deeds for others; helping them; taking care of them.

*Coaching Perspective:* "I love to help people and do nice things for them. I often reach out to my clients in special and caring ways that touch the heart."

### 12. Social intelligence (emotional intelligence, personal intelligence):

Being aware of the motives and feelings of other people and oneself; knowing what to do to fit into different social situations; knowing what makes other people tick.

*Coaching Perspective:* "I can easily understand and navigate people's feelings, needs, and desires (including those beneath the surface). People say I 'connect with respect,' the hallmark of my coaching."

## Justice

Civic strengths that underlie healthy community life:

### 13. Citizenship (social responsibility, loyalty, teamwork):

Working well as a member of a group or team; being loyal to the group; doing one's share

*Coaching Perspective:* "My clients always come first and think of me as being on their team. I love to be their partners in facilitating growth."

### 14. Fairness:

Treating all people the same according to notions of equality and justice; not letting personal feelings bias decisions about others; giving everyone a fair chance

*Coaching Perspective:* "It's not my agenda, but my client's agenda, that counts. I leave my personal opinions out of the equation as I seek to model fairness in all my dealings."

### 15. Leadership:

Encouraging a group, of which one is a member, to get things done while at the same time maintaining good relations within the group; organizing group activities and seeing that they happen

*Coaching Perspective:* "I model being a leader in my work and personal lives, and I demonstrate my leadership with my clients by encouraging and supporting them to be leaders in their lives."

## Temperance

Strengths that protect against excess:

### 16. Forgiveness and mercy:

Forgiving those who have done wrong; giving people a second chance; not being vengeful

*Coaching Perspective:* "I accept my clients right where they are and just the way they are. I am never judgmental and never suggest that my client is wrong; rather, I explore and appreciate the lesson in every situation."

### 17. Humility/modesty:

Letting one's accomplishments speak for themselves; not seeking the spotlight

*Coaching Perspective:* "Although I 'walk the talk' when it comes to my own path of development, I never call attention to myself or put myself up on a pedestal. We're all learners in my book."

### 18. Prudence:

Being careful about one's choices; not taking undue risks; not saying or doing things that might later be regretted

*Coaching Perspective:* "I love to design doable strategies with clients. I want my clients to be successful, and that requires setting goals that are specific, measurable, actionable, realistic, and timelined."

### 19. Self-regulation (self-control):

Regulating what one feels and does; being disciplined; controlling one's appetites and emotions

*Coaching Perspective:* "Silence is my friend. I love to take my time, to think through my thoughts and feelings, and then say just the right thing at just the right time to move my clients forward. I also am a role model for self-regulation in my personal wellness."

## Transcendence

Strengths that forge connections to the larger universe and provide meaning and purpose:

### 20. Appreciation of beauty and excellence (awe, wonder, elevation):

Noticing and appreciating beauty, excellence, and/or skilled performance in all domains of life, from nature to art, to mathematics and science, and to everyday experience.

*Coaching Perspective:* "My clients never cease to amaze me. I love to acknowledge their beauty, excellence, and skill. No matter where they are on the journey, there is always something to celebrate and relish."

### 21. Gratitude:

Being aware of and thankful for the good things that happen; taking time to express thanks

*Coaching Perspective:* "I bring an 'attitude of gratitude' to life that my clients usually pick up on and come to share. What a gift to be alive, to work together, and to learn new ways to experience well-being!"

### 22. Hope (optimism, future-mindedness, future orientation):

Expecting the best in the future and working to achieve it; believing that a good future is something that can be brought about

*Coaching Perspective:* "I always believe in my client's ability to become his or her best self. I know that self is in him or her, no matter what, and I love to bring it out in all its fullness."

### 23. Humor (playfulness):

Liking to laugh and tease; bringing smiles to other people; seeing the light side; making (not necessarily telling) jokes

*Coaching Perspective:* "There's no shortage of laughter when it comes to my coaching sessions. I love to make learning fun, enjoyable, and meaningful. We even learn to laugh at our mistakes along the way."

### 24. Spirituality (faith, purpose, religiousness):

Having coherent beliefs about the higher purpose and meaning of the universe; knowing where one fits within the larger scheme; having beliefs about the meaning of life that shape conduct and provide comfort

*Coaching Perspective:* "I see my clients as participating in a much larger narrative that includes the purpose and meaning of the universe. I love

to make that connection with my clients and to watch the mysteries unfold."

## Being Skills Tied to Strengths

When a coach is relying on their strengths, it is easier to access the being skills that support a strong, connected, and authentic coaching relationship. The good news is that strengths and being skills are connected:

*Mindfulness is related to:* self-regulation, bravery, integrity, perspective, citizenship, and social intelligence

*Empathy is related to:* social intelligence, self-regulation, love, curiosity, open-mindedness, perspective, forgiveness and mercy, and spirituality

*Warmth is related to:* vitality, love, social intelligence, kindness, gratitude, forgiveness and mercy, and humility/modesty

*Affirmation is related to:* appreciation of beauty and excellence, gratitude, kindness, hope, creativity, and perspective

*Calm is related to:* spirituality, bravery, integrity, open-mindedness, perspective, self-regulation, and prudence

*Zest is related to:* vitality, humor, gratitude, curiosity, love of learning, bravery, persistence, and appreciation of beauty and excellence

*Playfulness is related to:* humor, curiosity, creativity, vitality, hope, spirituality, and perspective

*Courage and authenticity:* integrity, bravery, social intelligence, fairness, and persistence

### References

Balick, M. J., & Lee, R. (2003). The role of laughter in traditional medicine and its relevance to the clinical setting: Healing with ha! *Alternative Therapies, 9*(4), 88–91.

d'Ansembourg, T. (2007). *Being genuine: Stop being nice, start being real.* Encinitas, CA: PuddleDancer Press.

Gallwey, W. T. (2000). *The inner game of work.* New York: Random House.

Gavin, J., & Moore, M. (2010). Body intelligence: A guide to self-attunement. *IDEA Fitness Journal, 7*(11), 42–49.

Harris, T. A. (2004). *I'm OK—you're OK.* New York: HarperCollins.

International Coach Federation. *Core competencies.* Retrieved March 25, 2014 from http://coachfederation.org/credential/landing.cfm?ItemNumber=2206&navItemNumber=576

Jordan, J. V., Walker, M., & Hartling, L. M. (Eds.). (2004). *The complexity of connection: Writings from the Stone Center's Jean Baker Miller Training Institute.* New York: The Guilford Press.

Langer, E., & Carson, S. (2006). Mindfulness and self-acceptance. *Journal of Rational-Emotive & Cognitive-Behavior Therapy, 24*(1), 29–43.

Leonard, T. (2002). *The fifteen frameworks: Hallmarks of the certified coach.* Retrieved November 1, 2008 from http://www.coachville.com/15frame.html

Peterson, C., & Seligman, M. E. P. (2004). *Character strengths and virtues: A handbook and classification.* New York: Oxford University Press.

Rath, T. (2007). *Strengths finder 2.0.* New York: Gallup Press.

Shapiro, S. L., Carlson, L., Astin, J., & Freedman, B. (2006). Mechanisms of mindfulness. *Journal of Clinical Psychology, 62*(3), 373–386.

Silberman, J. (2007). *Mindfulness and VIA signature strengths.* Retrieved April 26, 2015 from http://positivepsychologynews.com/news/jordan-silberman/20070327179

Wooten, P. (1996). Humor: An antidote for stress. *Holistic Nursing Practice, 10*(2), 49–56.

Zander, R. S., & Zander, B. (2002). *The art of possibility.* New York: Penguin Books.

# CHAPTER 4

# Expressing Compassion

*"If we only listened with the same passion that we feel about being heard."*

—HARRIET LERNER

## OBJECTIVES

**After reading this chapter, you will be able to:**

- Describe the impact of negative emotions on brain learning
- Describe how compassion supports self-determination
- Define empathy and discuss how it relates to compassion
- Describe an empathy protocol called nonviolent communication (NVC)
- Define the four key components of NVC: observations, feelings, needs, and requests

## How Coaches Handle a Client's Negative Emotions

Emotional states and the balance of negative and positive emotions have an enormous impact on the brain's capacity for learning. Coaches assist clients in developing optimal emotional states to support learning. The first step toward an "organized mind" is to tame an overdose of negative emotional frenzy that many people deal with daily (Hammerness & Moore, 2012). Negative emotions reduce the brain's ability to learn, to take in new knowledge and skills, by impairing the function of the prefrontal cortex, impairing access to working memory which is the raw material for creativity. This hampers curiosity, cognitive agility, and creative and strategic thinking.

A study of physician empathy (Hojat et al., 2011) concluded that patients whose physicians have high empathy scores were significantly more likely to have good control of blood sugar and cholesterol levels than physicians with low empathy scores. A coach's compassion makes an important contribution in helping clients handle their negative emotions. Most people, particularly those who have chronic diseases and feel badly about their personal contribution to a disease process, have a vocal inner critic, a voice that says "I can't do this," "I'm not good enough," and "I failed." Self-criticism is a potent source of negativity that depletes brain resources, making it hard to move forward.

When coaches radiate warmth, patience, and empathy, clients are better able to let go of the past, accept themselves, and feel self-compassion. It can be difficult for health professionals to be patient and empathetic when people are not making progress, and yet acceptance and empathy are essential if coaches are to help clients loosen the grip of negative emotions and self-talk.

Kristin Neff (2011), a psychologist studying self-compassion, who started a self-compassion movement, has studied the value of self-compassion as a method of processing negative emotions and suffering well. Self-compassion toward one's negative emotions leads to a softer, kinder motivation that improves the brain's ability to learn and change. Unfortunately, fear of failing and of being a failure is not an optimal source of motivation. In contrast, Neff's formula for self-compassion is an excellent guide for coaches; it starts with a mindful acceptance of negative emotions, followed by a heartfelt connection to others who share similar negative emotions, and, lastly, self-kindness, perhaps crossing one's hands over the heart area for a moment.

Goleman (2006) suggests that there are two types of emotional reactions: low road and high road. Low-road reactions occur automatically, such as when we hear a sudden noise in the night and our heart jumps. High-road reactions occur when we reappraise the situation, halting the further release of stress hormones, adrenaline and cortisol. Reappraisal dampens the overactive amygdala (the inner "uh oh" voice). When we reappraise events, we are more likely to remember the content of those events. When we can mindfully distinguish between an event and our interpretations of it, we are setting the stage for optimistic reappraisal. The reappraisal process is a matter of becoming aware of often unconscious interpretations, bringing relevant filters (values, beliefs, culture) to consciousness and introducing positive changes in our perspectives.

A task of a coach then is to support clients in making reappraisal a conscious, ongoing process. Optimistic reappraisals are important in building a client's internal resources. Reappraisal is not about suppressing emotions. In fact, suppression leads to higher levels of negative emotions and worsening disease symptoms. We are also vulnerable to errors and poor judgments when brain function is impaired by fear. The coaching conversation can bring this often unconscious process to the conscious mind, where it can be named and normalized. Calming the amygdala by naming the threat

enables more constructive activity in the problem-solving portion of the brain.

Fredrickson (2009) has shown that positive emotions improve attention, open-mindedness, creativity, and the ability to reach a strategic perspective. Furthermore, when we are able to attain and sustain a positive emotion to negative emotion ratio above 3:1, our level of resilience rises to enable our ability to adapt and change. Positive emotions are vital for brain learning in the moment and for a client's change success over time.

In each coaching session, coaches create an oasis for clients, one that is calm, mindful, undistracted, and positive. Coaches also help clients become more self-compassionate toward their negative emotions and inner critics and develop a level of positive emotions needed for curiosity and creativity, leading to new insights and possibilities. Coaches support clients in learning from their behavioral experiments to substitute curiosity for negative self-talk that can come from perceived failure.

## Exploring Self-Esteem

Self-esteem, the belief that one has value and worth as a person, or healthy self-respect, is an important basic need of human beings. It drives us to set a high bar for our achievements and then measure how well we are performing. In the right dose with a positive voice, it is a powerful source of productive motivation, spurring us forward to achieve great things. However, if performance falls short of one's internal standard, this drive can turn into an inner critic and a potent source of negative emotions. As a result, it can have a negative impact on one's ability to improve and maintain well-being.

The benefits of high self-esteem (Baumeister, Campbell, Krueger, & Vohs, 2003) include:

- Facilitates greater resilience through persistence in the face of challenge
- Leads to greater initiative
- Promotes leadership as those with higher esteem are more willing to speak up in group situations
- Has a relationship to feelings of happiness

Those with low self-esteem are "more prone than others to get sick or suffer other physical problems in connection with stressful daily events" (Baumeister et al., 2003, p. 27). Additionally, those with low self-esteem may benefit more from therapy than from coaching, and an appropriate referral should be considered.

However, there is a growing movement that the focus on fostering high self-esteem, largely emphasized in American culture in the middle of the 21st century, is also not all good. High self-esteem can also lead to more undesirable outcomes:

- Narcissism, coupled with aggression
- Increased focus on social comparison
- An inflated view of how others perceive the person with high self-esteem
- A willingness to be more critical of others
- A greater willingness to experiment with potentially risky health behaviors

If esteem is based on social comparison, rather than one's true sense of value, it is difficult to avoid a judgmental mindset, with a labeling of others as "good," "bad," "better," or "worse." Additionally, as others progress, the goals of the client would continually need to shift to keep up with the increased competition. When self-esteem is grounded in a client's comparison of self to others in their environment, their goals are driven by the success (or failure) of others rather than their own autonomous motivation.

Contingent self-esteem is experienced by people who are preoccupied with questions of worth and esteem and who see their worth as dependent on reaching certain standards, appearing certain ways, or accomplishing certain goals (Ryan & Brown, 2003). This is especially detrimental in the context of health and wellness behaviors and goals if clients are motivated by external drivers such as the desire to please and appear worthy to others rather than experiencing autonomous motivation.

When external factors are instigators of change, coupled with thoughts such as, "I want to please you" or "I will get in trouble if I don't do it," learning, creativity, and task performance are diminished. In coaching, if a client's self-esteem is dependent on the perception of the coach, the praise received from the coach, and the success of a goal, the pressure to meet expectations undermines success and lowers authentic enthusiasm.

## Self-Compassion: How to Suffer Well and Calm One's Inner Critic

Kristin Neff (2011) proposes that self-compassion includes three elements: self-kindness, a sense of common humanity, and mindfulness.

Self-kindness requires recognition that the human experience inevitably includes suffering, heartache, embarrassment, disappointment, and failure. When one practices self-kindness amidst such trials, one chooses to be gentle and forgiving rather than angry and self-critical. This kindness may need to be accompanied by a willingness to be vulnerable and be truly seen, imperfections and all.

Brené Brown (2012) suggests that shame is bred by harsh, self-critical judgment and is often kept hidden and secret to hide vulnerability. Fortunately, a good coaching relationship founded on trust and authenticity can help a client be more willing to experience and share vulnerability followed by self-kindness.

Having a sense that one is part of greater common human experience, rather than feeling isolated and individualized, also contributes to greater self-compassion. When a client is aware that he or she is likely not alone in experiencing such negative feelings, it becomes easier to accept those feelings.

Additionally, it is important to acknowledge that one's situation is impacted by the environment as much as it is by individual choice. The social context and environment (people, places, things) in which a client lives is equally important to address when considering behavior change and when identifying solutions for improved life experience.

Self-compassion involves openness to experiencing the full range of human emotions so that they are acknowledged and honored without suppression, avoidance, exaggeration, or rumination. The practice of mindfulness allows for a nonjudgmental and observational approach to one's thoughts and feelings.

## Self-Compassion Leads to Self-Determination

The benefits of self-compassion are numerous, especially related to a client's need for self-determination. First, experiencing a connectedness with others—acknowledging the interconnectedness of all humankind—supports one's most basic need for relatedness. When behaviors are driven by love, rather than fear, feelings of confidence and a sense of security are more likely to take hold. Frenzy is tamed, leading to a calmer heart and mind. When a client is calm, he or she is better able to make wise and intentional choices informed by emotional intelligence. Autonomy is supported when one is encouraged to be reflective and make choices in line with one's values, needs, and motivations. Better behavioral choices lead to an increased chance of success, or mastery experiences, which completes the circle in building confidence or a sense of competency for the next task.

## Nonviolent Communication: A Model for Expressing Compassion

Several useful tools for supporting compassion—both for the client and coach—can be found in the work of Marshall Rosenberg's framework of nonviolent communication. Since the 1960s, Rosenberg studied and developed a method for expressing empathy, a critical tool for experiencing compassion. Rosenberg's method, called NVC, takes a moment to learn and a lifetime to master (Rosenberg, 2005, 2006).

An empathetic connection can bring clients out, helping them acknowledge their feelings and needs, leading to a deeper awareness for the client and a more connected coaching relationship. Once this is accomplished, there's no limit to the constructive actions a client can take and the behavior changes they can make.

## Defining Empathy

Empathy is the respectful understanding of another person's experience, including his or her feelings, needs, and desires. It is not a prelude to the work of coaching; it is the work of coaching. Through the respectful and appreciative understanding of a client's experiences, the coach supports the client in expanding his or her awareness, creating openness, and facilitating change. All coaching relationships must begin with the premise that change is facilitated by a calm, safe, and judgment-free relational space in which people are free to honestly share their thoughts, feelings, needs, and desires without fear of judgment, ridicule, or pressure. This is especially true when clients experience a seemingly irresolvable conflict between what they want and where they currently are. The more a client feels "stuck" and unable to move, the more important it is for coaches to express empathy and to appreciate the discomfort of being on a fence.

Although coaches widely recognize the importance of creating such a generative relational space with clients, it is sometimes difficult to maintain a calm, safe, judgment-free posture in the face of health-risk behaviors. It becomes even more difficult when those behaviors persist in spite of a coach's best efforts to support self-responsibility and behavior change. As the coach, it is tempting to push the client hard to make change happen. It is important to remember, however, that this can actually interfere with empathy and provoke resistance to change.

People often confuse empathy with pity and sympathy. Understanding the distinction is important for coaches to learn. In the context of coaching, sympathy means identifying with someone's experience primarily on an emotional level. Sympathizing with someone means "I feel your pain" or "I share your joy." Sympathizing with someone who feels sad can make us feel sad. The same goes for every other emotion, both positive and negative. That's because emotions are contagious.

Although such "emotional contagion" is a dynamic shared by all animals (De Waal, 2006), using some of the same faculties as empathy, it doesn't involve listening with the whole being. Indeed, sympathy often interferes with listening because it turns our attention more toward our own feelings, needs, and desires than to those of the other. The result can be overlooking clients' needs and desires. That's why, although expressing pity and sympathy can help at times, it does not have the transformational power of empathy.

Pity is also not useful in the coaching relationship as it means grieving someone's experience, usually because of circumstantial hardships. For example, we may pity a starving child or an outcast member of society. Such sorrow can lead to charitable actions, such as giving assistance or showing mercy. Although helpful, these actions, which stem from viewing and relating to people as casualties, usually do not serve to empower them. A person who pities someone communicates in effect, "I feel sorry for you." That attitude undermines self-esteem and has no place in coaching. Few people like to be pitied, no matter how difficult the situation. Coaching comes from the framework of believing in the client's ability to learn from and grow in any situation. Pitying runs counter to this framework, implying fateful resignation.

Empathy is not about feeling sorry for someone; it's about understanding and respecting where someone is coming from. Empathy necessitates both emotional and cognitive awareness to appreciate a person's experience, to connect respectfully, and to give voice to what people may be feeling, needing, and desiring. Empathy requires full engagement and deep appreciation. There is no hurry or judgment in empathy; rather, there is a safe, calm, no-fault zone where people can discover and develop their truths. Whereas sympathy is typically not discretionary, welling up in us like an intruder in ways that are sometimes helpful and sometimes not, empathy treasures emotion as a guest. Its impact is to open clients up to significant learning, growth, and change.

When we are empathetic, we say in effect, "I respect your pain" or "I celebrate your joy." To do so, we recognize the emotion for what it is and appreciate what it has to teach us. This requires us to learn and use the language of empathy. Expressing empathy requires us to develop a different language. It necessitates conscious engagement of emotional intelligence and the intuitive dance of dialogue. It takes real mastery, especially when people are acting out their pain in hostile or destructive ways.

## COACHING CASE

**Wendy Well:** "I am having such a difficult time with my manager. I think I'm going to get fired from my job, and then how will I afford to eat all of the healthy foods we've been discussing?"

**Coach Carl with pity:** "Oh, you poor thing! It is just terrible the way your manager treats you! You should win a prize just for putting up with that!"

**Coach Carl with sympathy:** "I completely understand. I remember when I worked for someone just like that about 10 years ago. It is so frustrating to not be understood; I remember it just like it was yesterday, but I got through it and so can you."

**Coach Carl with empathy:** "It does sound like a difficult time, and I hear how worried you are while also really wanting to keep your positive momentum going."

## Expressing Empathy with Nonviolent Communication

The NVC model for expressing empathy assumes four important distinctions:

1.  Make observations, not evaluations. By limiting our descriptions to what can be perceived by the five senses (sight, hearing, taste, smell, and touch) in specific times and places, we stave off the tendency to judge, exaggerate, interpret, generalize, catastrophize, assume, or criticize. For example, "I failed to exercise last week" is an evaluation. "I went to the gym one time last week" is an observation.

2.  Express feelings, not thoughts. Many are in the habit of confusing thoughts and feelings. Although grammatically correct, none of the following sentences express feelings: "I feel like a failure," "I feel it is useless," "I feel that my boss is controlling," and "I feel inadequate." These are thoughts masquerading as feelings, and they are not useful in expressing empathy. NVC refers to them as "faux feelings."

3. Identify needs, not strategies. The distinction between universal human needs and specific strategies to meet those needs represents the crux of NVC. "Needs are more than the things we can't live without. They represent our values, wants, desires and preferences for a happier and more meaningful experience as a human. Although we have different needs in differing amounts at different times, they are universal in all of us," such as the need for competence, connection, safety, or love (New York City Nonviolent Communication [NYNVC], 2014). Although grammatically correct, none of the following sentences expresses universal needs: "I need you to stop at the store," "I need to work out every day," and "I need to get going on this project." These are strategies for meeting universal needs. They do not represent the needs themselves.

4. Make requests, not demands. Once we've become clear about the feelings and underlying needs, it's time to either confirm our understanding or agree on an action. Either way, NVC uses the language of request: "Would you be willing to tell me what you heard me say?" or "What agreements would you be willing to make with regard to exercise in the coming week?" It is important to respect both the autonomy of the person and the possibility of the moment.

Undergirding Rosenberg's method is an awareness of a causal connection between personal feelings and universal needs (i.e., "When universal needs are being met, people feel good. When they aren't being met, people feel bad."). These feelings and needs are often below the surface. No change is possible until and unless those needs are fully and respectfully recognized and expressed.

The lists in Table 4.1 are representative but not exhaustive (Tschannen-Moran, 2012).

More examples are included in *The Introduction to NVC* by Greg Kendrick (2007) and other summaries (e.g., Lamb, 2002). The point is not to memorize and quote such lists but to become aware of the generative value of connecting with people's feelings and needs in a calm, safe, and judgment-free way.

Whether clients show up for a coaching session with positive or negative energy, having their feelings and needs acknowledged can deepen connection and accelerate a session's progress.

Figure 4.1 depicts the NVC communication model. This model works equally well as both a format for expressing gratitude and celebration (when needs are being met) and for requesting understanding and agreements (when needs are not being met). Both dynamics are two sides of the same coin. To express feelings rather than thoughts and needs rather than strategies, it helps to have a robust vocabulary of feeling and need words.

The ambivalence a client may express in coaching is a universal experience in the process of change and should be welcomed and explored. Moving through the ambivalence can be a real challenge when clients are innervated by evaluations, thoughts, strategies, and demands. It helps to remember that behind every evaluation there is an observation, behind every thought a feeling, behind every strategy a need, and behind every demand a request. Becoming curious about underlying observations, feelings, needs, and requests is the key to developing and expressing empathy. Warm empathy is an incredible gift that can propel the conversation forward in unexpected and dynamics ways. As Carl Rogers once said, "Empathy feels damn good" (Rosenberg, 2005, p. 113). It is the key to building up the emotional capital that undergirds positive, health-promoting behaviors.

## The Role of Empathy for the Coach

An awareness of one's own feelings and needs is crucial if coaches want to be an empathic presence for their clients. A mindful coaching practice includes the intentional practice of acknowledging one's own feelings and needs outside of and within the coaching relationship. When coaches find it difficult to give empathy, it probably means they are not receiving enough empathy themselves. Both regular self-empathy and mutual empathy among significant others are essential practices for authentic coaching presence because a coach will not be able to be fully present with a client unless he or she can come to work free of distraction from beckoning unmet needs.

## Table 4.1  Needs-Related Feelings

| When Needs *Are Not* Being Met | When Needs *Are* Being Met |
|---|---|
| **Hostile**<br>Animosity, antagonistic, appalled, aversion, cold, contempt, disgusted, dislike, distain, hate, horrified, repulsed, scorn, surly, vengeful, vindictive | **Exhilarated**<br>Ecstatic, elated, enthralled, exuberant, giddy, silly, slaphappy |
| **Angry**<br>Enraged, furious, incensed, indignant, irate, livid, mad, outraged, resentful, ticked off | **Excited**<br>Alive, amazed, animated, eager, energetic, enthusiastic, invigorated, lively, passionate |
| **Annoyed**<br>Aggravated, bitter, cranky, cross, dismayed, disgruntled, displeased, exasperated, frustrated, grouchy, impatient, irked, irritated, miffed, peeved, resentful, sullen, uptight | **Inspired**<br>Amazed, astonished, awed, dazzled, radiant, rapturous, surprised, thrilled, uplifted, wonder |
| **Upset**<br>Agitated, alarmed, discombobulated, disconcerted, disturbed, disquieted, perturbed, rattled, restless, troubled, turbulent, turmoil, uncomfortable, uneasy, unnerved, unsettled | **Joyful**<br>Amused, buoyant, delighted, elated, ecstatic, glad, gleeful, happy, jubilant, merry, mirthful, overjoyed, pleased, radiant, tickled |
| **Tense**<br>Antsy, anxious, bitter, distressed, distraught, edgy, fidgety, frazzled, irritable, jittery, nervous, overwhelmed, pressured, restless, stressed out, uneasy | **Relaxed**<br>At ease, carefree, comfortable, open |
| **Afraid**<br>Apprehensive, concerned, dread, fearful, foreboding, frightened, hesitant, mistrustful, panicked, petrified, scared, suspicious, terrified, timid, trepidation, unnerved, wary, worried, reserved, sensitive, shaky, unsteady | **Curious**<br>Adventurous, alert, interested, intrigued, inquisitive, fascinated, spellbound, stimulated |
| **Vulnerable**<br>Cautious, fragile, guarded, helpless, insecure, helpless, leery, reluctant | **Confident**<br>Empowered, proud, safe, secure, self-assured |
| **Confused**<br>Ambivalent, baffled, bewildered, dazed, flustered, hesitant, lost, mystified, perplexed, puzzled, skeptical, torn | **Engaged**<br>Absorbed, alert, ardent, curious, engrossed, enchanted, entranced, involved |
| **Embarrassed**<br>Ashamed, chagrined, contrite, guilty, disgraced, humiliated, mortified, remorse, regretful, self-conscious | **Hopeful**<br>Expectant, encouraged, optimistic |
| **Longing**<br>Envious, jealous, nostalgic, pining, wistful, yearning | **Grateful**<br>Appreciative, moved, thankful, touched |
| **Tired**<br>Beat, burned out, depleted, exhausted, fatigued, lethargic, listless, sleepy, weary, worn out | **Refreshed**<br>Enlivened, rejuvenated, renewed, rested, restored, revived, energetic |
| **Disconnected**<br>Alienated, aloof, apathetic, bored, cold, detached, disengaged, disinterested, distant, distracted, indifferent, lethargic, listless, lonely, numb, removed, uninterested, withdrawn | **Affectionate**<br>Closeness, compassionate, friendly, loving, openhearted, sympathetic, tender, trusting, warm |
| **Sad**<br>Blue, depressed, dejected, despair, despondent, disappointed, discouraged, disheartened, downcast, downhearted, forlorn, gloomy, grief, heavy-hearted, hopeless, melancholy, sorrow, unhappy | **Peaceful**<br>Blissful, calm, centered, clear-headed, mellow, quiet, serene, tranquil |
| **Shocked**<br>Appalled, disbelief, dismay, horrified, mystified, startled, surprised | **Relieved**<br>Complacent, composed, cool, trusting |
| **Pain**<br>Agony, anguished, bereaved, devastated, heartbroken, hurt, miserable, wretched | **Content**<br>Glad, cheerful, fulfilled, satisfied |

From Tschannen-Moran, 2012.

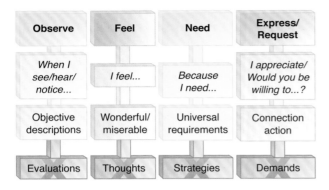

**Figure 4.1.** The NVC communication model.

By connecting deeply with their own feelings and needs or those of others (to the point of grieving when needs are not being met and celebrating when they are), coaches grow their empathy muscles and open the way for relational authenticity (Jordan, 2004). A masterful coach pays attention to develop the emotional intelligence needed to identify his or her own feelings and the needs driving those feelings.

*This being human is a guest house.*
*Every morning a new arrival.*

*A joy, a depression, a meanness,*
*some momentary awareness comes*
*as an unexpected visitor.*

*Welcome and entertain them all!*
*Even if they're a crowd of sorrows,*
*who violently sweep your house*
*empty of its furniture,*
*still treat each guest honorably.*
*He may be clearing you out*
*for some new delight.*

*The dark thought, the shame, the malice,*
*meet them at the door laughing,*
*and invite them in.*

*Be grateful for whoever comes,*
*because each has been sent*
*as a guide from beyond.*

—Rumi

## References

Baumeister, R. F., Campbell, J. D., Krueger, J. I., & Vohs, K. D. (2003). Does high self-esteem cause better performance, interpersonal success, happiness or healthier lifestyles? *Psychological Science in the Public Interest, 4*(1), 1–44.

Brown, B. (2012). *Daring greatly: How the courage to be vulnerable transforms the way we live, love, parent and lead.* New York: Gotham.

De Waal, F. (2006). *Primates and philosophers: How morality evolved.* Princeton, NJ: Princeton University Press.

Fredrickson, B. (2009). *Positivity: Groundbreaking Research Reveals How to Embrace the Hidden Strength of Positive Emotions, Overcome Negativity and Thrive.* New York: Crown Publishers.

Goleman, D. (2006). *Emotional intelligence.* New York: Bantam Books.

Hammerness, P., & Moore, M. (2012). *Organize your mind, organize your life.* Buffalo, NY: Harlequin.

Hojat, M., Louis, D. Z., Markham, F. W., Wender, R., Rabinowitz, C., & Gonnella, J. S. (2011). Physicians' empathy and clinical outcomes for diabetic patients. *Empathy, 86*(3), 359–364.

Humphrey, H. (2000). *Empathic listening.* In Empathy Magic Home Page. Retrieved October 16, 2008 from http://empathymagic.com/articles/Empathic%20 Listening%20'0061.pdf

Jordan, J. V., Walker, M., & Hartling, L. M. (Eds.). (2004). *The complexity of connection: Writings from the Stone Center's Jean Baker Miller Training Institute.* New York: The Guilford Press.

Kendrick, G. (2007). *An introduction to nonviolent communication (NVC).* In Celebrate Empathy with LifeTrek coaching. Retrieved October 16, 2008 from http://www.celebrateempathy.com/NVC_Intro.pdf

Lamb, R. (2002). *Communication basics: An overview of nonviolent communication.* Albuquerque, NM: Center for Nonviolent Communication.

Neff, K. (2011). *Self-compassion: The proven power of being kind to yourself.* New York: William Morrow.

New York City Nonviolent Communication. *Needs list.* Retrieved April 26, 2015 from http://www.nycnvc.org/needs.htm

Rosenberg, M. S. (2005). *Nonviolent communication: A language of life.* Encinitas, CA: PuddleDancer Press.

Rosenberg, M. S. (2006). The nonviolent communication training course: Home study course. Louisville, CO: Sounds True.

Ryan, R., & Brown, K. (2003). Why don't need self-esteem: On fundamental needs, contingent love, and mindfulness. *Psychological Inquiry, 14*(1), 27–82.

Tschannen-Moran, B. (2012). *Expressing Empathy with Nonviolent Communication.* Retrieved April 26, 2105 from http://www.schooltransformation.com/wp-content/uploads/2012/06/Expressing_Empathy.pdf

# CHAPTER 5

# Celebrating Our Best

> *"You are never given a wish without also being given the power to make it true."*
>
> —RICHARD BACH

## OBJECTIVES

**After reading this chapter, you will be able to:**

- Define positive psychology
- Define the role of positive psychology in the coaching relationship
- Name and discuss the five basic principles of appreciative inquiry (AI)
- Name and discuss each stage within the 5-D cycle of AI
- Describe the process of using AI to facilitate the development of a client's positive vision (or desired future) within a coaching session

## Positive Psychology

When Martin Seligman became president of the American Psychological Association (APA) in 1998, he had a vision of a new domain of psychology. Rather than mainly focusing on what ails the human mind (e.g., neurosis, anxiety, depression), Seligman proposed that psychology turn more of its attention to the conditions that enable people to flourish, to what makes people feel engaged, fulfilled, and authentically and meaningfully happy. This move-

ment became known as positive psychology and has delivered important applications for coaches as an evidence-based body of knowledge to support the process of behavior change and foster higher levels of well-being. This movement led Martin Seligman and his close colleague Christopher Peterson to complete a deep and thorough exploration of character strengths and virtues—understanding what is right with humans, not mostly what is wrong.

Strengths and strategies based in the principles of positive psychology, such as optimism and gratitude, are increasingly linked not just to greater mental well-being but also to greater physical well-being. Optimism is linked to better health outcomes, ranging from increased protection against cancer and cardiovascular disease to fewer colds (Seligman, 2011). Positive emotions are also correlated with higher longevity. Danner, Snowdon, and Friesen (2001) found that higher levels of positive emotion expressed in the autobiographies of young nuns (who used words such as "joy" and "thankful") were correlated to longer lives; those nuns lived up to 10 years longer than those who expressed lower levels of positive emotions and higher levels of negative emotions.

Chronic stress and the accompanying negative emotions have been shown to negatively impact health, whereas long-term positive emotions may prevent people from becoming ill, favorably affecting morbidity and mortality. Happy people are also more likely to engage in healthy behaviors. Positivity and health is a two-way street; good health generates positivity, and positivity generates good health, an upward spiral.

In her book *Positivity*, Barbara Fredrickson (2009) summarizes her 25-year research career focused on the study of positive emotions. Happiness is about focusing on a target for one's state of being—moment to moment, day to day, week to week, month to month. Data shows that 80% of people are below an optimal ratio of positive to negative emotions, which could be contributing to an epidemic of unhealthy lifestyle behaviors. With more positive emotions, people are healthier and have the resources to change and grow, bouncing back from adversity. Positive people flourish and find themselves on upward spirals. With fewer positive than negative emotions, people just survive, or even languish, falling into downward spirals.

## A New View of Positive Psychology

As the positive psychology movement matures, so does the perspective on its goals. In the early stages, there was strong focus on increasing one's happiness through positive emotions, engagement, and meaning: The end game was to feel good. Critics of the happiness movement suggest that there is more to life than happiness or just feeling good. For example, Gruber, Mauss, and Tamir (2011) suggest there is danger in the happiness movement because a life of thriving includes positive and negative emotions; in other words, a balance of emotions is important. Negative emotions serve an important role of informing us of dangers or unmet needs of ourselves or others.

Seligman (2011) then introduced the PERMA model of well-being with five components to expand on his initial thinking:

- Positive emotion
- Engagement
- Relationships

- Meaning
- Achievement

Fredrickson (2009) also goes beyond happiness to focus on flourishing. She contends that people who flourish not only feel good, but they also do good. They have a sense of purpose or calling, and they are highly engaged in life. Positive people give to others with their best possible selves to achieve their best possible futures. Fredrickson contends that the way to happiness is to flourish through cultivating positivity in order to be optimally resilient in the face of negativity. Hence, positivity is a necessity, not a luxury; it is an essential component of good health and well-being.

## How Does Coaching Generate Positivity?

An important mechanism of action for coaching is that coaches build positivity by helping clients define what makes them thrive, identify, cultivate, develop, and harvest more positive emotions and achieve important goals. These aspects of the coaching relationship keep the positivity spiral moving upward. Positivity is a key mechanism of action for resilience and life satisfaction (Fredrickson, 2009). Daily we are reminded that resilience in the face of minor or significant adversity is essential to human well-being, not just nice to have.

Coaching generates positivity by fostering the capacity, resources, and processes that are needed for successful change. Coaching helps clients identify what makes them flourish, building Fredrickson's (2009) top 10 positive emotions:

- Inspiration: connecting health and well-being to higher purpose and life meaning
- Hope: creating a vision of the future, identifying small steps forward that feel doable, and developing the experimental mindset of a scientist
- Pride: uncovering strengths and talents and appreciating success in meeting goals
- Interest: setting goals that are engaging and "a stretch" but not anxiety-producing
- Love: fostering trust, rapport, and connection with the coach and harnessing social support

- Awe: identifying inspiring role models and heroes
- Amusement: laughing at oneself and situations
- Joy: improving awareness and enjoyment of thriving
- Gratitude: appreciating life's gifts including challenges
- Serenity: stopping to savor moments of contentment

## Appreciative Inquiry (AI): A Tool for Celebrating the Best

AI is a philosophy as well as an approach for motivating change and enhancing well-being that focuses on exploring and amplifying the best in a person or situation. AI was developed initially in the late 1980s as a transformational change process for organizations and groups by David Cooperrider and his colleagues in the Department of Organizational Behavior at the Weatherhead School of Management at Case Western Reserve University in Cleveland, Ohio (Cooperrider & Whitney, 2005; Hammond, 1998; Whitney & Trosten-Bloom, 2003). It has since been adopted by many other disciplines, including positive psychology, sociology, and coaching.

AI does not focus on weaknesses and problems to fix; instead, clients are encouraged to acknowledge strengths and imagine possibilities in order to rise above and outgrow their problems. Given the value of building positive emotions, AI is a valuable coaching tool for uncovering and celebrating the best of what is and what could be.

Carl Jung (1962), a 20th century psychiatrist and founder of analytical psychology, describes the appreciative view of challenges in this way:

> The greatest and most important problems of life are all in a certain sense insoluble. . . . They can never be solved, but only outgrown. . . . This "outgrowing," as I formerly called it, on further experience was seen to consist in a new level of consciousness. Some higher or wider interest arose on the person's horizon, and through this widening of view, the insoluble problem lost its urgency. It was not solved logically in its own terms, but faded out when confronted with a new and stronger life-tendency. (p. 91f)

## Five Principles of Appreciative Inquiry

Building on Jung's insights, AI offers five principles (Fig. 5.1) that undergird its practice (Cooperrider & Whitney, 2005).

**Figure 5.1.** The five principles of AI lead to positive actions and outcomes.

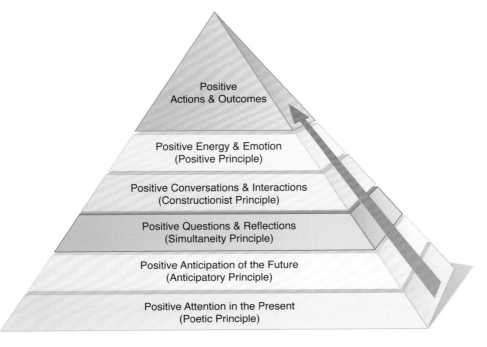

Positive Actions & Outcomes

Positive Energy & Emotion
(Positive Principle)

Positive Conversations & Interactions
(Constructionist Principle)

Positive Questions & Reflections
(Simultaneity Principle)

Positive Anticipation of the Future
(Anticipatory Principle)

Positive Attention in the Present
(Poetic Principle)

## The Positive Principle

*Positive actions and outcomes stem from positive energy and emotion.* The positive principle asserts that positive energy and emotion disrupt downward spirals, building the aspirations of people into a dynamic force for transformational change. Positive energy and emotions broaden thinking, expand awareness, increase abilities, build resiliency, offset negatives, generate new possibilities, and create an upward spiral of learning and growth. By identifying, appreciating, and amplifying strengths, people go beyond problem solving to make bold shifts forward. Demonstrating "why it's good to feel good," their actions become positively charged and positive outcomes are evoked (Fredrickson, 2003).

The positive principle asserts that positive actions and outcomes stem from the unbalanced force generated by positive energy and emotion. Newton's first law of motion states that objects at rest tend to stay at rest while objects in motion tend to stay in motion unless acted upon by an unbalanced force. Applying this law to human systems, the positive principle holds that the negative energy and emotion associated with identifying, analyzing, fixing, or correcting weaknesses lacks sufficient force to transform systems and propel them in new directions. At best, such root cause analyses will only correct the problems. At worst, they will cause a downward spiral.

## The Constructionist Principle

*Positive energy and emotion stem from positive conversations and interactions.* The constructionist principle asserts that positive energy and emotion are generated through positive conversations and interactions, leading to positive actions and outcomes. Through our conversations and interactions with other people, we create the realities in which we live. "Words create worlds" is the motto of AI in general and the constructionist principle in particular.

More than any of the other five principles, the constructionist principle makes clear the importance of the social context and environment in creating the present moment and changing future moments. Inner work and self-talk alone are not sufficient.

Different environments generate different truths and different possibilities. They even generate different dimensions of individual experience. As Rosamund Stone Zander and Benjamin Zander (2000) summarize the constructionist principle: "It's all invented! So we might as well invent a story or framework of meaning that enhances our quality of life and the lives of those around us" (p. 12). Clients can invent those stories and frameworks in conversations with their coaches.

## The Simultaneity Principle

*Positive conversations and interactions stem from positive questions and reflections.* The simultaneity principle makes the following claim: Conversations and interactions become positive the instant we ask a positive question, tell a positive story, or share a positive reflection. Positive questions and reflections are themselves the change we seek. They are not just a prelude to change; they are the change. They don't just begin a process that leads to a positive future; rather, positive questions and reflections simultaneously create a positive present. By shifting conversations and interactions in a positive direction, one can create a positive present. Positive conversations with a coach can create a positive world for the client.

The inquiries and reflections used in a coaching conversation are fateful. According to Jacqueline Bascobert Kelm (2005), "There are no 'neutral' questions. Every inquiry takes us somewhere, even if it is back to what we originally believed. Inhabiting this spirit of wonder can transform our lives, and the unconditional positive question is one of the greatest tools we have to this end" (p. 54).

## The Anticipatory Principle

*Positive questions and reflections stem from positive anticipation of the future.* The anticipatory principle asserts that when there is a positive anticipation toward the future, everything tilts in that direction. Positive anticipation of the future is a proleptic force that energizes the present. The word "prolepsis" literally means "a forward look."

The anticipatory principle asserts that it takes a specific, positive image of the future in order to impact the dynamics of the present. The more concrete and real the image, the more yearning and movement it creates. According to Warren Bennis and Burt Nanus (1985), "Vision is a target that beckons" (p. 89). Margaret Wheatley (1999) describes vision as a field (p. 53ff). As such, it is "a power, not a place, an influence, not a destination." It is best served, then, by imbuing the present with "visionary messages matched by visionary behaviors" (Wheatley, 1999). Anticipation becomes the hallmark and herald of change.

Equipped with a glimpse of what things look like at their best, a client will become more creative, resourceful, and resilient, finding ways to make things happen. The questions and reflections that a coach chooses flow from the coach's outlook in regard to the client. It is crucial that a coach adopts a sense of hope about the positive possibilities in a client's life.

### The Poetic Principle

*Positive anticipation of the future stems from positive attention in the present.* The poetic principle asserts that the more one attends to the positive dimensions of the present moment, the more positive the intentions for future moments will be. A focus on problems begets more problems; a focus on possibilities begets possibilities. With positive emotions, one's vision widens, and through this broadened mind, comes more flexibility, attunement to others, creativity, and wisdom (Fredrickson, 2013a, 2013b). Seeing and attending to the poetry of life is inspiring. It's not that problems disappear. Rather, other things become more important. Life's poetry evolves into a spiral of positive imagination.

Forming the base of a pyramid, on which all the other principles are built, the poetic principle connects hope with mindfulness and intention with attention. Becoming mindful of what adds richness, texture, depth, beauty, significance, and energy to life awakens life's magnificent potential. It's as though life becomes a work of great poetry, filled with hopeful meaning and forward movement toward positive growth and change.

## The 5-D Cycle of Appreciative Inquiry

The five AI principles have resulted in the development of a transformational change process that works with large groups as well as with individuals. Although the process has been described in various ways, the 5-D cycle (define-discover-dream-design-destiny) (Fig. 5.2) is the most common and easily remembered (Watkins & Mohr, 2001).

**Figure 5.2.** The 5-D cycle of AI helps guide clients through a transformational process to meet their goals.

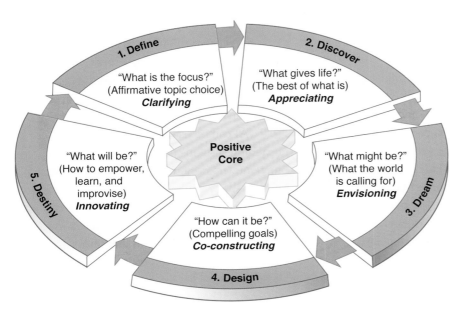

## Define

The process starts by securing an agreement between coach and client as to what the client wants to learn (topic choice) and how the client wants to learn it (method choice). The effectiveness of the AI process depends on the agreement being both clear and appropriate.

Some clients may not be ready, willing, or able to implement a strengths-based approach to transformational change. Get a sense of this by noticing how much they want to talk about their problems and their pains. Express compassion as an entry point to move the conversation forward. In the absence of forward movement after a reasonable amount of time, clients may make more progress with a therapist or counselor by developing ways to heal or process negative emotions and experiences.

## COACHING CASE

**Coach Carl:** "Great to reconnect with you again, Wendy. What is the most important topic for us to focus on in the 30 minutes we have together?"

**Wendy Well:** "Good question. By the end of our session, I would really like to have a game plan for managing my eating while I'm on vacation next week."

## Discover

Once the learning agreement is clear, the next step is to assist clients in discovering promising examples of their desired outcomes, both past and present. AI makes the assumption that in every person's life and situation, some things are always working, even though they may be buried and need to be unearthed. Life-giving examples, images, and stories that support the learning agreement can always be discovered.

To facilitate the discovery process, AI has developed an appreciative interview protocol that can be adapted and used by coaches at any point during the coaching process. It is particularly effective when clients are discouraged or stuck.

The AI protocol includes four discoveries:

1. *Best experience.* Even when people bring seemingly intractable challenges to the coaching session, it is important to encourage them to look at things through an appreciative frame and a light of curious wonder and interest. All situations have beauty and value, no matter how difficult. "Tell me a story about the best experience you have had dealing with such problems in the past" is an example of a way to reframe deficits into assets. Such stories assist clients in remembering that their lives are not problems to be solved but mysteries to be lived, and coaches can instantly marshal client concentration and energy. Although coaching is important work, a successful coach balances the serious nature of behavior change with the ability to make the process light and fun, eliciting a sense of adventure. The principles and practices of AI allow coaches to do just that. The coach who endeavors to stay positive, anticipate greatness, reframe reality, evoke insight, and share stories (the five principles) enables clients to experience coaching as bringing out the best in them rather than the worst. Through the processes of defining ambitions, discovering strengths, dreaming possibilities, designing strategies, and delivering the goods (the five practices) both coach and client alike have their spirits energized and lifted. The issues may be weighty, but the process of AI can lighten the load in the course of moving forward. Using humor, laughter, and playfulness in AI energizes the behavior change process so that solutions expand in scope, sustainability, and effectiveness.

AI can be used week after week in coaching sessions because people always have new experiences, values, conditions, and wishes to talk about. Instead of starting a coaching session by asking "So how did it go since the last time we met?," ask a more positive opening question that uses AI, such as "So what was your best experience (or your best learning experience) since the last time we met?" The coach may change the time frame or shift the focus but should always stay in a positive frame (New & Rich-New, 2003).

## COACHING CASE

**Coach Carl:** "Tell me about a time, perhaps on a vacation, when you were able to make healthy choices despite having temptations."

**Wendy Well:** "Oh, it's been a long time. You know, now that I think about it, I did pretty well a few weeks ago at my parents' surprise anniversary party."

2. *Core values.* AI emphasizes life-giving experiences, core values, generative conditions, and heartfelt wishes as it energizes clients to learn to make new contributions and to express new ways of being in the world. That is the fuel for destiny. The challenge is to enable clients not only to deliver on their promises but also to go beyond them. This happens when clients learn to experiment, innovate, and improvise so that they can take bigger, bolder, and better actions in the service of their dreams. Designs require continuous learning, dialogue, and updating in order to be fulfilled and fulfilling.

## COACHING CASE

**Coach Carl:** "So a few weeks ago, you were faced with some temptations at a party during what was a stressful, busy time, and you made healthy choices. Congratulations! What were the reasons that led you to make the choice to eat well then?"

**Wendy Well:** "One reason was that I wanted to have really great memories of the party—I'd been planning it for a year. I didn't want to think back on that evening and be upset by what I had chosen to eat."

3. *Generative conditions.* A masterful coach pays attention to the larger dynamics at play in a client's life rather than just the immediate goal or task. AI avoids fragmented interventions by recognizing the totality of the whole. For example, one of the more impactful consequences of the constructionist principle for coaching is in the area of self-improvement. People do not change by themselves, solely from the inside out; rather, change also happens from the outside in as we engage in conversation with others. Because self-improvement is influenced by relationships, it's important to use AI to open up the conversation to include environments, systems, communities, organizations, networks, movements, relationships, processes, policies, practices, structures, and resources.

## COACHING CASE

**Coach Carl:** "You relied on your strengths of self-regulation and perspective to make choices that you knew you would feel good about later. What else supported you in being healthy that day?"

**Wendy Well:** "Since I was planning and really managing the party, I didn't think I'd get to eat much during it anyway. So about two hours before it began, I had my husband bring me a grilled chicken salad from a restaurant around the corner. That kept me from feeling too hungry later in the night."

4. *Three wishes.* "Tell me about your hopes and dreams for the future. If you found a magic lamp and a genie were to grant you three wishes, what would they be?"

The purpose of these discoveries is to boost the energy and strengthen self-efficacy of clients through the vivid reconnaissance of mastery experiences. The more direct, personal, and relevant the mastery experiences, the greater their positive impact on a client's motivation for and approach to change.

## COACHING CASE

**Coach Carl:** "Great planning! As you think about your vacation, what three wishes do you have for creating ideal memories with no regrets?"

**Wendy Well:** "I want to enjoy my food, slowly savor each bite, and not regret anything I've eaten at the end of the day."

The discovery phase of AI can be viewed as the most important phase in the coaching session. It elevates self-confidence and lays the foundation for all that follows. That's why it's so important to not rush through the discovery process in order to get to goal setting. The simultaneity principle makes clear that asking appreciative questions is not a prelude to the work of coaching; it is the work of coaching. Inquiry into what happens when the client functions at his or her best is transformational in and of itself. It not only forms the basis for change, it is the change in which they seek.

### Dream

Once clients have discovered the best of "what is," it is time to encourage them to envision the best of "what might be." The discoveries of the last phase are used to create a dream that is grounded in the client's history, as it expands the client's potential. Moving beyond the level of three magical wishes to the level of realistic but provocative propositions about the future, the dream will be even larger than the client would otherwise have imagined without the discovery phase having been done.

In the dream-making process, AI encourages the use of both left brain and right brain activities. The poetic principle goes beyond the limitations of analysis by using stories, narratives, metaphors, and images to make dreams come alive.

Several considerations impact the dream-making process. The first is the question of a calling: What is life calling a client to be or become? The second is the question of energy: What possibilities generate excitement for a client? The third is the question of support: What is the positive core that supports a client?

Don't be lured into creating provocative possibilities for a client. "The client finds the answers. The client finds the answers. The client finds the answers." Encourage clients to generate their own possibilities by thinking outside the box without regard to consequences. After clients have accessed their own creative resources, coaches may or may not offer to put additional ideas on the table for consideration. In every instance, the client retains the choice in creating the dream, design, and destiny.

When the dream becomes a target that beckons and an anticipatory field that surrounds and supports a client's best self, it is time to move on to design.

## COACHING CASE

**Coach Carl:** "Those three wishes are very clear. I'm curious—what is your deeper goal here? How does this fit into your larger life goal?"

**Wendy Well:** "Gosh, if I can live with no regret on vacation—a time when people usually let their guards down and have no rules—I can do anything in the 'real world.'"

### Design

The design phase of the AI process gives the dream legs by working to align the client's infrastructure with the dream. Clients are asked to make proposals and set goals as to how the dream would manifest itself in terms of habits, procedures, systems, technology, roles, resources, relationships, finances, structures, and stakeholders. What would shift if a client's infrastructure were aligned with his or her dream? Describing those shifts in detail is the fundamental work of the design phase.

It is important to make the design phase as detailed and personal as possible. Encouraging clients to make commitments, offers, and requests with a close horizon, perhaps a one- or two-week deadline, is relevant to both this and the final phase of the process.

- Commitments represent actions that clients promise to take in response to the requests of others.
- Offers represent actions that clients volunteer to take.
- Requests represent actions that clients seek from others in order to successfully implement the design.

## COACHING CASE

**Coach Carl:** "It sounds like your dream for vacation fits well into your bigger dreams for yourself. Would you like to begin to create a plan for your vacation?"

**Wendy Well:** "Absolutely."

**Coach Carl:** "What is the commitment you are ready to make?"

### Destiny

The purpose of AI is to elevate both the positive energy and self-efficacy of clients in order to assist them in realizing their destinies. It is not just a feel-good process; it is also an action process that makes dreams come true and makes dreaming intrinsic to the client's way of being in the world. By developing an "appreciative eye," clients learn to make the 5-D cycle their preferred approach to problems and opportunities in order to fulfill their destinies. They learn to continuously innovate their way to even higher levels of performance and life satisfaction.

## The Value of Appreciative Inquiry in Coaching

AI is a valuable tool for energizing, motivating, and mobilizing a client toward behavior change. It starts with the presumption that anything is possible (the constructionist principle) and then employs a methodology (the 5-D cycle) to help clients make it happen, thus elevating both self-esteem and self-efficacy. The increases in positivity and self-efficacy lead naturally to the dream, design, and destiny phases. When done well, the mounting energy and motivation for change generated by the discovery phase of the AI process are palpable. The anticipatory consideration of best experiences, core values, generative conditions, and heartfelt wishes through a vivid investigation of past and present increases the client's readiness, willingness, and ability to move forward into the future. "Now what?" and "How do we get going?" are the operative questions of the later phases. AI generates an expansive upward spiral that enables clients to successfully mount the behavior change pyramid. By going through the 5-D cycle multiple times, clients and coaches create dreams and designs beyond those initially imagined possible.

The AI protocol is a great place to start, especially when clients do not have a clear focus. It can kindle the embers of desire until the fire is burning bright. It can also support specific client learning and development. For example, instead of asking clients for a generic best experience story related to health and wellness, ask them for a best experience story that is specifically related to their positive visions (or desired futures). Such targeted learning from a positive frame can dramatically accelerate the behavior change process.

AI requires clients to use a mixture of analytic activities and creative activities. It is not enough to encourage clients to identify and commit to SMART goals (goals that are specific, measurable, actionable, realistic, and timelined). No matter how well-crafted the strategy, a purely analytic approach will fail if it is not supplemented by a process that engages the client's heart and stirs the client's imagination. SMART goals must also be compelling goals.

To this end, AI encourages clients to be creative by imagining, articulating, and designing their dreams for the future. Clients can use pictures, images, metaphors, art, movement, music, and/or stories (the poetic principle). The more creative the dreams, the better when it comes to making the case and generating the energy for change. Clients often enjoy the invitation to use their whole selves in the development of their dreams and designs for the future. There is no end to what they will come up with once they have the permission and encouragement to get creative (e.g., changing body position, drawing pictures, modeling clay, standing on tables, stepping over lines, writing poetry, ringing bells, singing songs, stretching muscles, controlling breath, telling stories, shouting affirmations, and imagining visualizations).

It is tempting to think that the outcome of using AI in coaching is a clear plan with detailed next steps. Although that is often the case, it is not the only or ultimate outcome. AI sets in motion an appreciative and innovative approach to lifelong learning. The destiny phase of the 5-D cycle has been described as going back around the cycle again and again in perpetuity. When clients learn how to define-discover-dream-design, as their way of being in the world, they end up realizing their destiny as they grow into their best selves. The 5-D cycle is not just a tool or technique for coaches to master, it is also—and most importantly—a way of living. By using and sharing AI with our clients, we empower lifelong upward spirals of personal and organizational development.

## But Really, What About Problem Solving?

It is the nature of the human mind to zoom in to look at what's not working, to notice, analyze, and solve problems. But that does not necessarily make it the best or most effective strategy to use. Indeed, tackling problems head on often provokes discouragement and resistance rather than fostering encouragement and readiness to change. This insight

is what led to the development of AI as a way of solving problems through the back door. Instead of tackling problems head on, AI assists clients in outgrowing problems through engaging in new and stronger life urges. In the process, problems that once seemed overwhelming and intractable lose their energy and sometimes even fade from view.

When working on client challenges with the AI framework, keep the following in mind:

## "You Have What It Takes to Succeed"

This is the posture of great coaching. If a coach does not believe in the ambitions and innate abilities of their client, it will negatively impact progress toward improved health and well-being. If a coach questions a client's desires and capabilities or does not believe he or she has what it takes to succeed, then it may be time to refer that client to another coach or helping professional.

## "My Certainty Is Greater than Your Doubt"

Great coaches come from this framework, but know that it is better to not directly make this argument to their clients. We provoke skepticism and resistance when we attempt to persuade clients that they can do something. We evoke confidence and movement when we stay with clients in the muck until they become clear about where they want to go, how they want to get there, and how they will generate the energy. Great coaching communicates a calm energy of confidence on which clients can build and from which they can learn.

## Speak the Truth in Love

If the definition of love includes "mutual care," it is important for coaches to bring this to the coaching relationship, especially in times of challenge. Without falling into the trap of arguing for change, it is important for coaches to honestly share what they see. If there is an elephant in the room and the client fails to notice it, it may be time for a client to hear the coach speak the truth in love. The energy for change is not created by naive or delusional self-appraisals. Clients who are not fully engaged, being honest with themselves, following through on their promises, working hard, and/or making progress may benefit from coaches reflecting these perceptions. Returning to the 5-D cycle is another way to encourage the client to move forward.

## Use Appreciative Inquiry to Handle a Client's Self-Sabotage

Avoid "wrestling" with clients who are not meeting their goals or following through on their promises week after week. Instead, use the 5-D cycle to make sure the goals and promises are exciting to the client and appropriately scaled to the client's capacity. Setting goals or making promises because they would be "good for the client" represent something the client "should" do and will generally fail over time, as is the case with goals that are designed to "please the coach." Setting goals or making promises which stretch the client's capacities must include appropriate, capacity-building strategies in order to be stimulating and effective. If after employing these strategies and not provoking resistance the coach still cannot assist a client to move forward, it may be true that the client is experiencing challenges that that go deeper than coaching can resolve. If so, it may be time to make a therapeutic referral.

## Coach the Client and the Environment

Designing environments to be supportive of a client's goals and promises is essential for client success. A strength-based approach to coaching does not work in isolation from a client's environment. Indeed, the design phase of AI makes clear the importance of whole system frameworks, including various internal/external and individual/collective dynamics. In the design phase of the 5-D cycle, the role of the coach is to make sure that a client does not overlook or ignore any aspect of the system. For example, the client may need to learn new skills, modify his or her environment in order to eliminate triggers, or gather social support. Friends, colleagues,

and relatives can provide emotional support, practical support, partnering, or listening ears.

Examples include:

- Exercising with someone
- Phoning someone daily or several times a week
- Reporting progress regularly to someone
- Eating with someone and gaining support for health-supporting choices
- Sharing goals, food logs, and exercise goals
- Joining a gym with a friend or spouse
- Having a spouse watch the kids while exercising

## Stay in a Positive Frame

Again, it is human nature to selectively notice and focus on problems. We have a negativity bias; we scan the environment for negative information, even if the negative event only happens once (Hanson, 2009). That's why news headlines get our attention when they focus on tragedies, terrorism, and scandals.

The coach begins with empathy, appreciating the power that fear and anxiety have over a client. Coaches create a safe coaching environment where clients can relax rather than being distracted by scanning the environment for danger and other negativity. Fear also presents an opportunity to educate clients about brain science so they understand that the brain is wired to be instinctively afraid, even if the negative emotions are out of proportion with the real threat.

The 5-D cycle of AI shifts the spotlight away from train wrecks and onto the positive aspects of the past, present, and future. When clients drift into an analysis of past or present failures, it is important to gently but firmly bring them back to an appreciative frame. Acknowledge the problem, and then invite them to look at it from a different perspective. Two possible questions to ask to make the shift from a traditional problem-solving approach are "How did this make a positive contribution to your development?" and "How else would you describe this situation?" When the coach adopts a positive frame, a client will eventually follow. By using the generic AI interview protocol, it is possible to quicken the interest of clients in the life-affirming and life-giving dimensions of their own experiences.

### It Is "Trial and Correction" Not "Trial and Error"

Trial and correction, rather than trial and error, underlies AI. The process is analogous to the nearly universal human learning experience of learning how to walk. Those first few tentative baby steps occur after months of watching other people walk upright. These role models awaken in toddlers the desire and ambition to walk, and at the appropriate developmental moment, begin to encourage them. They stand the toddlers upright, hold their hands, and move them forward. With outstretched arms, they cheer and cajole until the brave youngsters take their first unsupported steps.

No one teaches toddlers how to walk with step-by-step instructions. They don't have the biomechanics explained to them. They figure it out for themselves in a gradual process of trial and correction. After the first steps, toddlers inevitably fall down. This does not provoke criticism or condemnation. No one takes it as a failure. On the contrary, toddlers are cheered on, encouraged to try again and again until they master the skill.

Enabling clients to loosen up and experiment with different strategies without the fear of failure is the essential work not only of AI but also of coaching. Brainstorming provocative possibilities using the 5-D cycle is one way to make that happen. Such possibilities can be provocative in part because it is unknown whether or not they will work. Only time will tell through the process of trial and correction.

Sharing stories with each other is a great way to incorporate the richness of "trial and correction" into coaching sessions. Stories have a way of inducing people to discover and discern their own meanings and movement. Like a toddler watching people walk, when we listen to each other's stories,

our ambition awakens, evoking more robust motivation for change.

### Acknowledge Success

Clients easily lose sight of their progress when they have setbacks or don't reach their goals as quickly as they wish. Keep reminding them of past progress, no matter how much or little they have made. For example, "Three months ago, you couldn't walk a mile" or "Before we started, you wouldn't have even noticed that the restaurant meal was high in calories. You're more conscious of those issues now, and your body is used to lighter food. That is a big step!" Remember, masterful coaches champion their clients in each and every conversation.

## Using Appreciative Inquiry to Transform the Coaching Relationship

Because coaching promotes client development within a learning partnership, it is important for coaches to solicit feedback from clients. Many clients need permission to honestly share their feelings and wishes about the coaching experience. The appreciative interview protocol can be modified to encourage honest sharing and elicit feedback through a positive frame. For example, at periodic intervals during the coaching program, the following inquiries could be used:

- "What's the best experience you have had so far through the coaching process?"
- "What are the values you most often see me modeling as a coach?"
- "What conditions have most helped you reach your goals and move forward?"
- "If a genie were to grant you three wishes regarding our coaching relationship, what would they be?"

Feedback solicited through this appreciative frame is quite different from criticism. By focusing on positive, life-giving experiences, values, conditions, and wishes, both coach and client are empowered to be honest and to make the coaching relationship as productive and as enjoyable as possible by motivating change that focuses on exploring and amplifying strengths.

## References

Bennis, W., & Nanus, B. (1985). *Leaders: The strategies for taking charge.* New York: Harper & Row.

Cooperrider, D. L., & Whitney, D. (2005). *Appreciative inquiry: A positive revolution in change.* San Francisco: Berrett-Koehler Communications.

Danner, D. D., Snowdon, D. A., & Friesen, W. V. (2001). Positive emotions in early life and longevity: Findings from the nun study. *Journal of Personality and Social Psychology, 80,* 804–813.

Fredrickson, B. L. (2003). The value of positive emotions: The emerging science of positive psychology is coming to understand why it's good to feel good. *American Scientist, 91,* 330–335.

Fredrickson, B. L. (2009). *Positivity: Groundbreaking research reveals how to embrace the hidden strength of positive emotions, overcome negativity, and thrive.* New York: Crown.

Fredrickson, B. L. (2013a). *Love 2.0: Finding happiness and health in moments of connection.* New York: Penguin.

Fredrickson, B. L. (2013b). *Love 2.0: How our supreme emotion affects everything we feel, think, do and become.* New York: Hudson Press.

Gruber, J., Mauss, I., & Tamir, M. (2011). A dark side of happiness? How, when, and why happiness is not always good. *Perspectives on Psychological Science, 6*(3), 222–233.

Hammond, S. A. (1998). *The thin book of appreciative inquiry.* Bend, OR: Thin Book.

Hanson, R. (2009). *Buddha's brain: The practical neuroscience of happiness, love and wisdom.* Oakland, CA: New Harbinger.

Jung, C. G. (1962). *The secret of the golden flower: A Chinese book of life* (R. Wilhelm, Trans.). San Diego, CA: Harcourt Harvest Books.

Kelm, J. B. (2005). *Appreciative living: The principles of appreciative inquiry in personal life.* Wake Forest, NC: Venet.

New, B., & Rich-New, K. (2003). *Looking for the good stuff.* Cape Canaveral, FL: Clarity Works!

Seligman, M. (2011). *Flourish: A visionary new understanding of happiness and well-being.* New York: Free Press.

Watkins, J. M., & Mohr, B. J. (2001). *Appreciative inquiry: Change at the speed of imagination.* San Francisco: Jossey-Bass/Pfeiffer.

Wheatley, M. J. (1999). *Leadership and the new science.* San Francisco: Berrett-Koehler Communications.

Whitney, D., & Trosten-Bloom, A. (2003). *The power of appreciative inquiry: A practical guide to positive change.* San Francisco: Berrett-Koehler Communications.

Zander, R. S., & Zander, B. (2000). The art of possibility. New York: Penguin Putnam.

# CHAPTER 6

# Harnessing Motivation to Build Self-Efficacy

*"Whether you think you can or can't, you're right."*

—HENRY FORD

## OBJECTIVES

**After reading this chapter, you will be able to:**

- Describe the difference between controlled and autonomous motivation
- Define motivational interviewing (MI) and discuss how it is integrated into coaching
- Name the key MI tools, including a variety of reflective listening statements and the use of rulers to evoke readiness to change
- Define and discuss four sources of self-efficacy

## Harness Motivation to Build Self-Efficacy

This manual opened with a simple description of coaching: Coaching is a growth-promoting relationship, which elicits motivation, increases the capacity to change, and facilitates a change process through visioning, goal setting, and accountability; at its best, this relationship leads to sustainable change for the good. This chapter focuses on two of these key elements—"elicits motivation" and "increases the capacity to change."

You may also recall that in Part 2 of Chapter 1 on coaching psychology, we proposed four coach-

ing mechanisms of action. We described two of these mechanisms as the twin engines of change—self-motivation ("I want to do it") and self-efficacy ("I believe I can do it"). We explored how these two mechanisms build on self-determination theory. In this chapter, we explore other science-based constructs, theories, and models, which add to the discussion of motivation and self-efficacy in coaching. We draw further from self-determination theory and address the four principles of MI. We explore the four sources of self-efficacy defined in social cognitive theory (SCT). We also weave in references to the early research on life purpose and meaning, nonviolent communication (NVC), appreciative inquiry (AI), and flow theory. The next chapter on the transtheoretical model identifies other change processes that are related to motivation and self-efficacy.

## What Does It Mean to be Motivated?

Motivation is the energy that can drive one to:

- Start a new habit or learn a new skill
- Take steps toward a goal
- Focus on making a habit or learning a skill toward a goal

- Sustain a habit or skill
- Appreciate and savor goal achievement

However, not all types of motivation are created equal, and not all strategies for uncovering motivation increase a client's drive and commitment to change.

## Controlled Motivation

Motivation may come from an external source with the good intentions of motivating a client to make critical behavior changes or to change unhealthy thinking. External sources of motivation can have the best outcomes in mind for a client while pushing, strongly encouraging, or even demanding "compliance" in behavior change. Words such as "should," "must," and "have to" imply an external standard or expectation that relates to self-respect and self-esteem. "I am a good or bad person depending on whether I do a behavior," a form of internal compliance is implied, and this is in contrast to a heartfelt desire for the behavior's outcome.

### COACHING CASE

**Controlled Motivation**

**Coach Carl:** "OK, Wendy, I'm pretty concerned about the fact that you are still smoking. You've been so great about making great strides in your health over the last few months, but this is an area that hasn't improved and is concerning. I know you'd feel so much better and proud of yourself if you made some progress in this area, and I am certain that you can do it! Also, are you aware of your employer's new incentive program? If you commit to participate in the "Smoke Freedom" program and stay active in it for three months, you'll get a $50 gift card. Wouldn't it be great if we could say we accomplished this?"

**Wendy Well:** "Well, OK, I guess I can give it a try."

When clients respond to external motivation with changes in behavior, they are most likely driven to comply by a desire to please another or get this person's approval or respect. They may also be reacting to the fear of consequences for not doing so. Simply put, long-term behavior change does not reliably result from force, facts, or fear (Deutschman, 2007). This is why, for example, many patients with heart disease often require multiple procedures that could have been prevented if lifestyle changes had been made.

Unfortunately, although external motivation sometimes leads to compliance, it also leads to defiance rooted in a person's need for autonomy, the deep need to march to one's own drummer rather than comply with another's wishes. When one acts in compliance with another's desires, a sense of autonomy is jeopardized. The need for autonomy is so fierce that people may resist and rebel against expert advice on healthy lifestyle change just to preserve autonomy. Parents of teenagers know this phenomenon all too well, and it is universal across the lifespan to resist being told what to do, from the "terrible twos" to elders who are hanging onto their independence for as long as they can.

Edward Deci (2013), co-founder of self-determination theory, suggests that although it is possible to get people to behave in healthy ways through seduction or coercion or through the use of financial incentives, the behavior will only last as long as the incentives are there. This means that an expert advisor or employer delivering an external source of motivation may not lead to self-generated motivation and may even eventually provoke resistance and defiance, making people less likely to engage than without the external motivator.

## Autonomous Motivation

How does a coach support a client in unleashing his or her own motivation without the use of force, facts, fear, or good old-fashioned cheerleading? The answer is tapping into the client's autonomous motivation.

Autonomous motivation is about behaving with a full sense of volition, interest, and choice. When people are autonomously motivated, they control their choices, and they are acting in ways they find interesting, important, better, or of deep value (Deci, 2013).

Deutschman (2007) cites the work of Dr. Dean Ornish, a professor of medicine at the University of California at San Francisco and founder of the Preventive Medicine Research Institute. Ornish (2002) also recognized the importance of a higher quality motivation which took into account the psychological, emotional, and spiritual dimensions of change. In his work with patients who had had a heart attack, he noticed that patients would be "compliant" with the "doctor's orders" only for a few weeks after the event and out of fear (Ornish, 2002).

However, in the long term, patients stopped thinking about their mortality, denial would return, and they would return to their unhealthy lifestyles. So Ornish (2002) took a different tact; rather than motivating patients with the "fear of dying," he supported them in considering a new vision, focused on the "joy of living" and the benefits that come with living. He recognized that joy is a more powerful motivator than fear.

When behavior change is intrinsic, clients experience pleasure—it's fun, challenging, and interesting. This kind of motivation can be present-focused, savoring its impact in the here and now and how good it feels to have made healthy choices at the end of a day. Or it can be future-focused, with the client knowing that the change will lead to a better future, energizing him or her to make the world a better place, stepping closer to his or her "best self," and recognizing that a bigger reward comes after the behavior is sustained.

According to Deci (2013), the benefits to people who experience high autonomous motivation are big. They include:

- New and positive behaviors persist longer.
- They are more flexible and creative.
- Performance improves.
- People experience more enjoyment in making changes.
- People have better physical health and higher quality personal relationships.

Autonomy is a core human drive as Deci and Ryan (2002) have taught us; we are wired to dislike being told what to do. Clients perform best when they are free to make an autonomous choice. This is good news because people also assume responsibility for their health when they act autonomously. The U.S. healthcare system is designed to be top-down and authority-led, putting the patient in the passenger seat while the healthcare provider sits in the driver's seat, determining the agenda and delivering advice and education. This deprives a patient of the opportunity to take charge and drill down to find a heartfelt source of motivation. The coaching model, which starts by eliciting autonomy, can help shift this dynamic in the healthcare system.

When there is an awareness of the importance of the need for autonomous motivation, positive results follow. For example, Deci (2013) cites a smoking

## COACHING CASE

**Autonomous Motivation**

**Coach Carl:** "Wendy, what is on your mind for our session today? You've raised a few topics in previous conversations—a desire to get more rest and your interest in quitting smoking. Would you like to discuss either of these, or is there something else you want to talk about today?"

**Wendy Well:** "Well, I've been procrastinating on the conversation about smoking for months now. I know my employer is really getting strict with insurance and that my being a smoker is going to have an impact."

**Coach Carl:** "So, on one hand, your employer is encouraging all employees to quit smoking. On the other hand, you have a choice in the matter. Is this something you want to discuss today, or is there something more important to you?"

**Wendy Well:** "Quitting smoking is actually pretty important to me. It's just so hard to quit, and frankly, I can't stand being told what to do."

**Coach Carl:** "It is frustrating when you feel you don't have control. Let's look at the ways you are in control here. What about quitting is important to you?"

cessation study that looked at the degree to which medical staff supported patient autonomy. By meeting patients' fundamental psychological needs, the staff supported patients in becoming more autonomously motivated; the patients then perceived themselves as more competent in their ability to quit smoking.

Coaches engage in undistracted listening and reflecting with an open, mindful, and curious mindset rather than preaching and prescribing, which triggers resistance and even defiance. Clients are often taken aback when they connect for the first time with their own heartfelt desire for change—it's not about pounds on a scale, it's about unleashing clients' desires to improve their health so that they have the resources they need to live the lives they most want to live.

## Motivational Interviewing: A Model for Increasing Motivation and Self-Efficacy

MI is a counseling methodology developed over the past 30 years initially as a new approach to the treatment of addiction. MI methods support the eliciting of autonomous motivation, encouraging a client to find his or her own reasons to change. It involves pro-change talk and avoids triggering of change-resistance talk, which can cause the client to resist being told what to do.

In coaching, the more clients make their own case for change (pro-change talk), the more likely they are to actually make changes. Conversely, the more coaches make the case for change, the more likely it is that client resistance will increase and the motivation for change will decrease.

MI aims to increase autonomous motivation for change with the following strategies developed by MI founders Rollnick and Miller (2012):

1. Engaging: developing growth-promoting and relationship-building strategies that support the client's autonomy
2. Focusing: helping clients develop more clarity around their values and goals
3. Evoking: generating a connection to the client's autonomous motivations and drives

4. Planning: designing action plans that support the building of self-efficacy

MI explicitly avoids the top-down expert approach in favor of assisting patients to make their own best decisions about why, what, how, and whether to change (Pantalon et al., 2013). Below we explore the four MI principles, integrating other theories and models that support and extend these principles.

## Motivational Interviewing Principle 1: Engaging

MI starts with the premise that pro-change talk is facilitated by a calm, safe, judgment-free relational space in which people feel secure in honestly sharing their thoughts, feelings, needs, and desires without fear of judgment, ridicule, or pressure. This is especially true when clients experience a seemingly irresolvable conflict between good reasons to not change and good reasons to change. The more a client feels "stuck" and unable to move forward, the more important it is for coaches to express empathy and to validate and appreciate the discomfort. And, the more labeling, assessing, telling, and demanding that the coach does, the less engaged the client will become.

MI holds that efforts such as pushing, nagging, prodding, enforcing, and insisting that clients make change are usually counterproductive because they encourage resistance talk rather than change talk, which hinders the advancement of the client's agenda and the work of coaching in general. To summon empathy and leave promotional efforts behind, it helps to recognize risky behaviors, like smoking, as expressions of a client's unmet needs. No change is possible until and unless those needs are fully and respectfully recognized, expressed, and appreciated.

## Rolling with Resistance

MI holds that a client's resistance talk says more about the approach of the coach than about the client's readiness to change. One way to show support for client autonomy is to "roll with resistance." The fact is clients do not resist change, but they resist being changed. Marshall Rosenberg (2005) describes resistance-creating approaches as life-alienating communication, noting that the following forms of communication can increase resistance and interfere with empathy:

- Moralistic judgments
- Diagnostic labels
- Enemy images
- Guilt trips
- Making demands
- Denying choice or responsibility
- Rewards and punishments
- Making comparisons

Holley Humphrey (2000) notes that the following communication patterns also interfere with empathy, whether they are intended to be constructive or not. That's because they come more from pity and sympathy than they do from empathy.

- Advising: "I think you should …" "How come you didn't …?"
- Educating: "This could turn into a very positive experience for you if you just …"
- Consoling: "It wasn't your fault, you did the best you could."
- One-upping: "That's nothing; wait until you hear what happened to me."
- Storytelling: "That reminds me of the time …"
- Shutting down: "Cheer up. Don't feel so bad."
- Interrogating: "When did this begin?"
- Commiserating: "Oh, you poor thing."
- Explaining: "I would have called but …"
- Correcting: "That's not how it happened."

All of these approaches increase the likelihood of resistance talk. The use of empathy, inquiry, and reflection increase the likelihood of change talk. Empathy makes the relational field between client and coach both safe and interesting, opening the door to new possibilities and facilitating change. Instead of arguing with clients or fighting fire with fire, empathy helps redirect and thereby diffuse the energy of resistance in constructive ways.

Learning to roll with resistance is an essential skill in masterful coaching. Coaches pushing back against resistance can increase resistance and can move clients backward in their readiness to change. When a coach feels the temptation of the "righting reflex" to confront resistance directly, such as by arguing, diagnosing, fixing, or any other communication pattern that fosters resistance, it is important to take a deep breath; extend self-compassion for one's need for the client to change; and then respectfully explore the client's underlying feelings, needs, and desires. The more curious we become about those underlying feelings, needs, and desires while suspending our own judgments, interpretations, assumptions, evaluations, and agendas, the greater the chance of developing a life-giving connection and facilitating change talk.

The followings perspective shifts may assist coaches in rolling with resistance:

- *From client resistance to an external desire to connection.* The more a coach tries to get a client on board or seek compliance, the more a client resists change. In contrast, the more a coach seeks to respectfully understand the client's experience, the more open a client becomes.
- *From authoritative expert to inspiring confidence.* The more a coach claims to know what's best for a client, the more likely resistance will be provoked. In contrast, the more the coach believes in a client's ability to learn, the more confident a client becomes.
- *From causes to capacities.* The more a coach digs for causes of problems, the more trouble is dug up. The more a coach and client collaboratively search for capacities, the more engaging the change process becomes.
- *From counterforce to counterbalance.* The more forcefully a coach argues against ambivalence and for change, the more a client will push back. The more a coach counterbalances client ambivalence with appreciative awareness of the good reasons to not change, the more change talk is generated.

Once an empathic connection is made, MI encourages coaches to use open-ended questions, reflective listening statements, as well as a variety of rulers to develop awareness of the gap that may exist between present behavior and important personal goals or values. The coach should not point out the discrepancies, which can feel judgmental. That can trigger resistance to behavior change. Rather, clients should be encouraged to notice the discrepancies for themselves. When they do, they will experience new feelings, become aware of new needs, and express new desires. Exploring discrepancies with empathy and curiosity can help clients to become more open and motivated to change.

## Open-Ended Inquiry

Along with other models used by coaches, MI leverages the full value of open-ended inquiry. Recall that all of the questions in the discovery phase of AI (related to best experiences, core values, generative conditions, and heartfelt wishes) are open-ended. Such questions allow clients to take an active role in the coaching session as they explore both the positive and negative impacts of their behaviors.

Some examples of open-ended questions that evoke change talk are:

- What is the best experience you have had with your desired future behavior?
- What concerns do you have about your current behavior?
- What values do you seek to live by in your life?
- How might your desired future behavior lead to benefits in the future?
- How might your current behavior lead to problems in the future?
- What changes would you like to make in your routine? (Miller & Rollnick, 2012)

As clients tell their stories and give expression to their full experience, the discrepancies that become self-evident may seem overwhelming. If this happens, the coach can best help a client by expressing empathy and appreciation for the good reasons leading to ambivalence.

Because open-ended inquiry encourages the client to process his or her experience and talk more than coaches, ideally more inquiries in a coaching session are open-ended than closed-ended.

## Perceptive Reflections

Reflective listening statements function like mirrors, enabling clients to see themselves in new ways and improve both motivation and capacity for change. Timely and provocative reflections (empathy for unmet needs, amplification of topics that might improve motivation and confidence) are at the heart of the MI model. MI uses more reflective listening statements than questions of any type. That's because questions tend to generate left brain thinking-dominated responses, whereas reflections tap into emotions and needs. Additionally, a series of questions all in a row can make people feel interrogated. The ideal ratio of reflections to questions over the course of a session is about 2:1. This is a good rule of thumb for coaching too.

Empathy reflections, or "empathy guesses" as they are referred to in the language of NVC, are particularly valuable for expressing empathy. "When we are thinking about people's words, listening to how they connect to our theories, we are looking at people—we are not with them" (Rosenberg, 2005). The key to being "with" a client is to be wholly present with them by listening for the feelings that they are expressing and the needs that are being met or unmet.

## Motivational Interviewing Principle 2: Focusing

The second principle of MI is to enable a focused exploration of the discrepancies between a client's stated values and goals and their current behaviors. This principle is narrower than the focus of a typical coaching session in which a coach and client collaborate to determine the focus and agenda for the session. Rather, this principle is about more narrowly directing the focus on the gap between a client's present situation and their values and goals. This can be appropriate if offered to a client first as one of several options and he or she chooses to proceed to explore this discrepancy as the next best step.

## Developing Discrepancy

Exploring a decisional balance, the pros and cons of a particular change, is a helpful tool in assisting clients to think through whether they are ready, willing, and able to make a change. Open-ended questions and reflective listening statements encourage clients to thoroughly consider the pros and cons of change. What are the costs and benefits of not changing? What are the costs and benefits of changing? A decisional balance discussion helps clients more fully appreciate the sources of their autonomous motivation (costs of not changing, benefits of change) and what is required to build confidence (finding possible strategies to deal with the benefits of not changing and the costs of changing).

Physician and MI expert Richard Botelho (2004) uses a quantitative rating system (Fig. 6.1), along with the decisional balance conversation in his tool for promoting change talk and increasing motivation. Coaches can use this tool during coaching sessions.

A coach can either help a client focus on one column at a time (e.g., focusing first on all of the reasons to stay the same) or use a technique called mental contrasting where the client would alternate—first identify a reason to stay the same and then a reason to change, and back and forth (Oettingen & Gollwitzer, 2010).

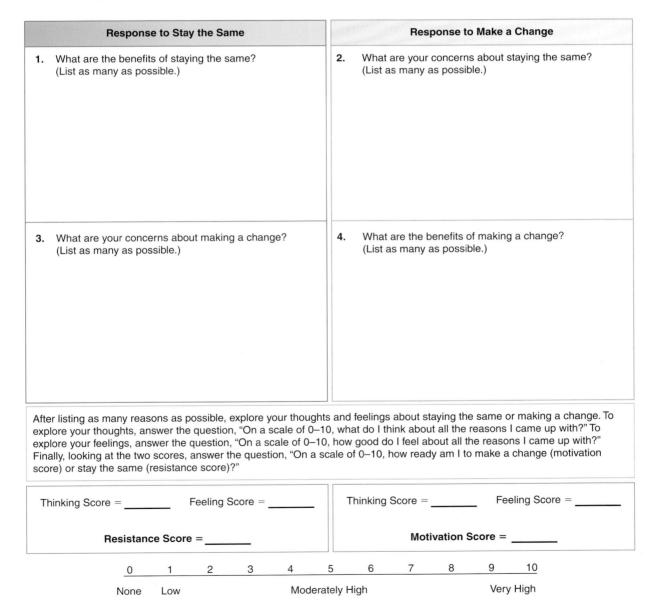

**Figure 6.1.** Tool for developing discrepancy.

Clients are first asked to list the benefits and concerns about not making or making a change. Once the lists are generated, clients are asked to rate on a scale of 0–10 (with 10 being the highest and 0 being the lowest) what they think and feel about their lists. After looking at the thinking and feeling scores, clients are then asked to assign composite scores to their levels of resistance and motivation to change.

## Perceptive Reflections for Developing Discrepancy

Four powerful reflections used by MI practitioners to develop discrepancy between the desired future and current behaviors are simple, amplified, double-sided, and shifted-focus reflections. Each can be used in conjunction with an NVC-style empathy reflection, addressing the client's feelings and needs.

### Simple Reflections

These reflections are like the images seen in a flat mirror. A simple reflection paraphrases and restates what clients are saying, using their own words without exaggeration, interpretation, or distortion. The impact of such simple reflections can be surprisingly powerful.

## COACHING CASE

**Wendy Well:** "I don't have time to exercise. My friends and my spouse don't either!"

**Coach Carl's simple reflection:** "It seems that you, your friends, and your spouse don't have time to exercise."

**Wendy Well:** "That's true, except for one of my friends who is an avid runner. I don't know how he does it!"

**Coach Carl's empathy reflection:** "When you say you have a friend who is an avid runner, it sounds like you are impressed and may be curious, wondering how he manages to find the time."

### Amplified Reflections

These reflections are like the images seen in a convex or concave mirror. They maximize or minimize what clients say in order to evoke disagreement from them in the direction of change talk. By reflecting an increased or decreased intensity of a client's perspective, magnifying both the affect and the outcome, clients may react quickly with new insights and reasons to change. To avoid being manipulative, the coach should use statements only in the service of client-generated goals. To avoid being mocking or patronizing, the coach should deliver such statements in charge-neutral terms.

## COACHING CASE

**Wendy Well:** "I don't have time to exercise. My friends and my spouse don't either!"

**Coach Carl's amplified reflection:** "I hear you saying that you don't know anyone close to you who has time to exercise and that it feels impossible for you to fit exercise into your schedule."

**Wendy Well:** "It's not impossible for me to exercise. It's just hard to find the time. Once in a while I do manage to exercise, and I know there are people out there who exercise regularly, so maybe I could figure out a way."

**Coach Carl:** "Sounds as though you are curious and feeling a little energized about finding a way to exercise more regularly, learning from the experience of others."

### Double-Sided Reflections

These reflections are like the images seen in trifold mirrors; they reveal multiple perspectives at the same time. By encouraging clients to look at different facets, perhaps comparing a current resistant statement with a prior readiness statement, they gain perspective and make different decisions as to if and how they want to move forward.

## COACHING CASE

**Wendy Well:** "I don't have time to exercise. My friends and my spouse don't either!"

**Coach Carl's double-sided reflection:** "I hear you saying that you don't have time to exercise and that your friends and spouse don't either. But I've also heard you say that exercise makes you feel better and that regular exercise would be good for your energy and health."

**Wendy Well:** "That's the problem. I want to exercise, and it does make me feel better, but it cuts into my time with family and friends. If I could figure out how to do both, perhaps I could make exercise stick."

**Coach Carl:** "It sounds like you are feeling discouraged because it's hard to meet your needs for both exercise and connection, and it would be worthwhile to find a way."

### Shifted-Focus Reflections

These reflections are like the images we see in a periscope. They redirect our attention away from a resistance-provoking subject in order to focus on another area. Once change talk begins in that area, the resistance-provoking subject can be reconsidered with more success.

It is important to note that when a coach employs amplified and empathy reflections, it is a guess as to what will stimulate change talk and what feelings and needs may live behind a client's words, body language, or tone. Whether the guess is right or wrong does not matter. What matters is the integrity of the intention to generate change talk and to connect with honesty and empathy. Such attempts generate appreciation, awareness, and movement in the client. Because such reflections often bring to the surface strong feelings and deep needs, it's important to stay with the language of empathy until clients feel acknowledged and heard.

## COACHING CASE

**Wendy Well:** "I don't have time to exercise. My friends and my spouse don't either!"

**Coach Carl's shifted focus reflection:** "This sounds challenging, so little time to exercise. I'm wondering about the dance class you started with your partner. You were doing pretty well with that; I remember you saying that you were enjoying the classes."

**Wendy Well:** "Yes, that's the best decision I've made in quite a while. No more sitting in front of the TV on Thursday nights! It's been great to do something active together. We may even add a second night to the schedule."

**Coach Carl:** "It sounds like you are feeling happy with dancing and the time with your partner because it's meeting your needs for both physical activity and connection."

## Motivational Interviewing Principle 3: Evoking

The third principle of MI centers on uncovering a client's reasons for change. Encouraging the client to explore their autonomous "why" behind a behavior change, especially with an orientation toward the future, can create the energy needed for a shift. As Rumi said, "What you seek is seeking you."

## The Role of Meaning in Motivation

One's sense of purpose and meaning can also be an important foundation for reasons for change. The quest for meaning is the key to mental health and human flourishing, including overcoming adversity. By nature, humans are meaning-focused, motivated by the desire to understand the world in which we live and to search for something out there that demands our devotion (Frankl, 2006).

In his research, Paul Wong (1987), found that having a sense of meaning, life purpose, and life control were predictors of psychological and physical well-being. Wong concludes that meaning is necessary for healing, resilience, optimism, and well-being. An interesting new research direction concerning purpose led to the Boyle et al. (2012) finding that people with Alzheimer's disease who had a strong sense of life's purpose were less affected by brain plaques and tangles than were people with Alzheimer's disease without a strong sense of purpose. Even though their brains were similarly physiologically diseased, something about having "purpose" prevented the disease from fully manifesting in cognitive decline.

Coaches help clients examine the larger value and purpose behind any desired change, mining the past for lessons learned, the present for what contributions the change could make to performance and life purpose, and the future related to potential contributions to causes beyond self.

## COACHING CASE

**Wendy Well:** "Quitting smoking is actually pretty important to me. It's just so hard to quit, and frankly, I can't stand being told how to do it by non-smokers."

**Coach Carl:** "It is frustrating when you feel you haven't discovered yet how best to quit. Let's look at what is under your control here. What about quitting is important to you?"

**Wendy Well:** "Well, it would get my employer to stop nagging me."

**Coach Carl:** "That sounds like a good outcome. I'm curious about other outcomes that matter even more. What else do you see that would be an immediate benefit?"

**Wendy Well:** "I'd probably lose this nagging cough that keeps me from getting a good sleep."

**Coach Carl:** "And what else?"

**Wendy Well:** "My coworkers wouldn't look at me like I have the plague."

**Coach Carl:** "It sounds like that is hurtful for you. What do you wish was happening?"

**Wendy Well:** "I feel a bit like an outcast around them. I miss out on some conversations and fun when I'm taking smoke breaks during lunch, for example."

**Coach Carl:** "You really want to feel like you aren't missing out on any of the opportunities to connect with them. You want to feel included."

**Wendy Well:** "Yes, that's it."

**Coach Carl:** "And beyond the workplace, which is just one aspect of your life, what would it mean to you to be free of smoking?"

## Examining Motivation with Rulers

MI readiness and confidence rulers are useful tools for the exploration of motivation to change (Fig.6.2).

These scoring rulers enable clients to think out loud and quantify qualitative topics that are hard to pin down—their readiness, willingness, and ability to change. To evoke willingness, MI asks clients to rate the importance of making a change right now.

The coach might ask, "On a scale of 0–10, how important would you say it is to change your _____ at this time?"

With all three rulers, it is valuable to explore with a client: "What led you to not pick a lower number?" "What would help you get to a higher number?" Open-ended questions such as these, followed by perceptive reflections, can evoke change talk and support behavior change.

## Motivational Interviewing Principle 4: Planning

The MI principle of planning involves collaborating on an action plan supported by increasing self-efficacy. Let's explore the broader topic of self-efficacy next before addressing the MI planning principles.

## Self-Efficacy

Self-efficacy, the belief that one has the capability to initiate and sustain a desired behavior, is one of the most important outcomes of coaching in combi-

To evoke a willingness rating, MI asks clients to rate how important is it to make a change right now. The coach might ask, "On a scale of 1–10, how important is it to you to change your _____ at this time?"

**Figure 6.2.** Readiness, willingness, and confidence rulers.

**Willingness Ruler**

0   1   2   3   4   5   6   7   8   9   10

Not important          About as important          Most important
at all                 as everything else          thing in my life

To evoke an ability rating, MI asks clients to rate how confident they are at being able to make a change right now. The coach might ask, "On a scale of 0–10, how confident are you that you can change your _____ at this time?"

**Confidence Ruler**

0   1   2   3   4   5   6   7   8   9   10

I do not think I will     I have a 50% chance     I will definitely
achieve my goal           of achieving my goal    achieve my goal

After exploring importance and confidence, it may be helpful to ask directly about a client's readiness to change right now. The coach might ask, "On a scale of 0–10, how ready are you to change your _____ at this time?"

**Readiness Ruler**

0   1   2   3   4   5   6   7   8   9   10

I am not ready          I am almost ready          I am very ready
to change               to change                  to change

nation with improvements in self-image (becoming one's best self) and lasting mindset and behavior change. A goal of coaching is for clients to achieve and sustain the goals that brought them into coaching and to feel confident in their ability to attain new goals in the future, navigating challenges well as they arise. In other words, clients should be able to learn how to learn and change so that they can move on from a coaching partnership in self-directed, motivated, and confident ways.

## Social Cognitive Theory (SCT)

A primary resource for understanding self-efficacy is SCT, officially launched in 1986 with the publication of Albert Bandura's book, *Social Foundations of Thought and Action: A Social Cognitive Theory.* Simply put, SCT asserts that human behavior is determined by three factors which interact with each other in dynamic and reciprocal ways: personal factors (such as what one believes and how one feels about what one can do), environmental factors (such as support networks and role models), and

behavioral factors (such as what one experiences and accomplishes). SCT is named as such because it emphasizes the primacy of cognitive processes in constructing reality and regulating behavior.

Psychologist Mihaly Csikszentmihalyi (2003) believes that self-efficacy increases when one experiences flow—when the challenge of the task and the skills to accomplish it are high and close to equal. When one is engaged in a task that is mismatched with one's skill, efficacy decreases and anxiety increases.

Self-efficacy is impacted by all three factors (personal, environmental, and behavioral), and masterful coaching works to align those factors. Bandura (1994, 1997) indicates that it is important to pay attention to four sources of self-efficacy: physiological/affective states, verbal persuasion, vicarious experiences, and mastery experiences. Combined with other bodies of knowledge including the self-determination theory, the transtheoretical model of change (TTM), AI, NVC, MI, and positive psychology (including positive emotions, flow, and strengths), Bandura's work on self-efficacy complements the coaching toolbox by bringing a unified framework to these different but overlapping theories.

## Physiological/Affective States—Cultivating Eustress, Minimizing Distress

Nothing is more personal than one's body and feelings, both of which can interfere with self-efficacy. That's why it's so important to assist clients in becoming physically and emotionally comfortable with rather than intimidated by the prospect of change. The reasons for change become motivational only when they engage the whole person, including the person's physical sensations and emotional reactions, which can signal met or unmet needs. Simply put, how people feel about the prospect of change impacts their self-efficacy. If they have butterflies in their stomachs or a dry throat while approaching a task, for example, they are more likely to have low self-efficacy than when approaching a task feeling relaxed and confident. That may seem obvious, but the cause-and-effect relationship goes both ways; physiological states affect self-efficacy and vice versa, and coaches work to elicit both.

If stress is defined as stimulation, then distress represents either too much or too little stimulation. As noted earlier, the former provokes anxiety, whereas the latter produces boredom. Both are distressing, and in the extreme, both can generate negative health impacts.

Eustress, literally defined as "good stress," occurs in the flow zone. We find ourselves engaged but not overwhelmed, in control of our experience but not bored. This is the sweet spot that coaches seek to hit with clients, both during the coaching session—challenging clients to stretch their thinking and feeling while being affirmative and empathetic to avoid distress (Rosenberg, 2005)—and after the coaching session, as clients actively pursue their visions and goals.

Giving respectful attention and understanding to physiological/affective states, both during and between coaching sessions, can assist coaches and clients in finding that sweet spot. For example,

during coaching sessions, coaches can offer empathy reflections to elicit and connect with what clients may be feeling and needing in the moment. Coaches can also ask clients to change body position, breathe rhythmically, move their hands, walk around, trace a labyrinth, look at an object, draw pictures, play music, or connect in other ways with their physiological/affective states as different actions are being contemplated and reviewed.

The same is true for the coach's own physiological/affective states because they often mirror what a client is feeling and needing. The more aware coaches become of their own sensations and feelings in the moment as a coaching session progresses, the more on-target coaches become with their questions and interventions.

Getting clients to pay attention to their physiological/affective states between coaching sessions is equally vital in assisting clients in moving forward. Noticing and understanding what's happening on an emotional level while clients are experimenting with behavior changes can assist clients in discovering the things that fill them with or drain them of energy. Self-efficacy increases as clients do more of the things that fill them with energy. Coaches help clients set aside the pursuit of things out of a sense of obligation or the idea that they should in favor of doing things out of a sense of choice and the feeling that it is what they value and want. When the locus of control shifts from the external to the internal frame, clients find more energy, motivation, and greater confidence to change.

## Verbal Persuasion— Evoking Change Talk

Many different environmental factors impact self-efficacy; two of the most important are the things people say to us (verbal persuasion) and the things people do around us (vicarious experience). Verbal persuasion is not about wearing the "expert hat" and telling clients what they should do. That typically generates both resistance and resentment. Wearing the appreciative hat and stimulating a client to discover what they can do, however, is an entirely different matter. Inputs such as these tend to enrich life and generate movement as clients become persuaded that they have what it takes to initiate and maintain a desired behavior.

However, the more coaches try to persuade clients of what they should do, the more resistance coaches evoke, which decreases readiness to change. To assist clients to become persuaded without provoking resistance, coaches communicate confidence in the ability of clients to reach their vision and achieve their goals. When that confidence is heartfelt, sincere, and based on client strengths, it helps bolster self-efficacy. Although it may take time and many such verbal inputs from a variety of socially interactive phenomena, client inertia can be overcome. Put simply, the coach's belief in a client increases a client's belief in himself or herself.

It is the work of the coach not only to assist clients with the decisional balance of weighing pros and cons but also to support clients in acquiring the belief that they have what it takes to move forward and that life will support them in wonderful ways once they get started. As we have mentioned, Dave Buck of CoachVille frames the persuasive work of coaching in the terms, "My certainty is greater than your doubt." Such persuasion involves all aspects of being, including the cognitive, emotional, physical, and spiritual domains. It hinges on the track record and credibility of the coach and the quality of the coaching relationship.

Albert Bandura (1997) would caution against inauthentic, or unrealistic, persuasion suggesting that "cheerleading" for behaviors that aren't realistic undermines a client's progress and the coach's efforts. Bandura's recognition that verbal persuasion must be appropriately scaled reflects the basic insight of the transtheoretical model's stages of change as well as Csikszentmihalyi's work on flow. Masterful coaches dance with their clients to set appropriate, stage-specific challenges and to identify the relevant skills to be learned over time. When this happens, the coaching relationship can remain indefinitely productive because there are always new challenges to tackle and new skills to learn. AI is an especially powerful framework and process for assisting clients to become persuaded

that they have what it takes to do what they want to do. By evoking the stories of their best experiences and exploring their core values, strengths, generative conditions, and heartfelt wishes, clients become empowered to dream, design, and deliver their destinies.

When clients express resistance, the TTM, NVC, and MI models are invaluable. Resistance may come from the coach's inaccurate assessment of a client's readiness to change, setting a challenge that does not match the client's capacity, or formidable internal and external obstacles. Resistance may also develop when coaches speak from the expert position, telling clients what they "need," should, or "have" to do to reach their goals. MI uses many tools to avoid provoking resistance, including expressing empathy, silence, attentiveness, open questions, as well as reflective listening statements. These MI tools have the ability to shift the client from resistance talk to change talk, thus increasing the client's perceived self-efficacy.

Bandura (1994) notes that it is far easier to discourage someone with our words than it is to encourage them. The wrong words spoken at the wrong time can undermine confidence and produce disappointing results. Wearing the expert hat can overwhelm and intimidate rather than empower and inspire. It's better to listen and remain silent than to push the wrong buttons in our attempt to get things moving.

## Vicarious Experiences— Observing Similar Role Models

The world's first commercial bungee jumping took place in November 1988 off the Kawarau Bridge in Queenstown, New Zealand. The 43-meter drop continues to attract thousands of visitors each year who find it fascinating to watch the process of someone deciding to take the plunge. When people arrive, they first go to the viewing platforms, one high and the other low. They watch people of different genders and ages get strapped in and dive off the bridge into the gorge. With each successive jump, some become more interested, open, and confident. They develop the belief that "I can do that too." Their self-efficacy increases by the vicarious experience of watching the others.

Such experiences are yet another vital environmental factor when it comes to self-efficacy. The more opportunities people have to witness and relate to others who are doing what they want to do, the more likely it is that they will initiate and sustain that behavior themselves (Deutschman, 2007).

Sharing and telling stories are other ways for clients to have efficacy-building, vicarious experiences. Coaches can encourage clients to tell stories of others who have successfully handled their current goals and challenges. Coaches can also tell stories from their own life experiences and the experiences of others with whom they have worked or known. The more positive change stories coaches and clients share together, the more vicarious experiences come into the coaching conversation—and the more self-efficacy grows.

It's better to encourage clients to find their own stories of vicarious experience rather than to tell stories, but both can come into play over the course of a coaching conversation. When coaches tell too many stories, it can sound either boastful ("Look what I did!") or demanding ("All these people got their acts together! Why can't you?"). When stories are told judiciously, however, as part of the give and take of the coaching session, they serve as powerful tools to generate the energy for change.

If and when clients are unable to come up with their own stories of vicarious experience, coaches can encourage them to do research and field studies. To use the analogy of bungee jumping, coaches can assist clients in finding a platform from which to watch others do what they want to do. When this happens, their self-efficacy is likely to increase. The more success stories clients have in their repertoire and the more they tell those stories to their coaches and to others, the more likely it becomes that they will see themselves as able to achieve their desired outcomes.

That's especially true if the stories describe people similar to themselves. The greater the perceived similarity, the greater the impact a vicarious experience will have on self-efficacy. Why do some people decide to jump off the Kawarau Bridge while others demur, even though everyone has the same vicarious experience? It may have to do, in part, with how closely one identifies with those who take the plunge.

## Mastery Experiences— Successful, Perseverant Efforts

The fourth SCT factor, the behavioral factor, is both the most powerful source and the ultimate outcome of self-efficacy. What we actually accomplish ourselves does more than anything else to cultivate successful, perseverant effort. As the old saying goes, "Nothing breeds success like success." Conversely, "Nothing breeds failure like failure." Understanding this dynamic, masterful coaches assist clients in achieving quick wins and then staying on the winning path from week to week. Positive outcomes lead to increased self-efficacy, whereas negative outcomes lead to decreased self-efficacy. That's why mastery experiences can be viewed as both cause and effect when it comes to self-efficacy.

That's as true in coaching as it is in other areas. Masterful coaches do a better job of dancing with their clients than do uncertain or insecure coaches. As a result, masterful coaches generate better results and attract more clients—both of which serve to enhance their sense of self-efficacy as coaches. Instead of a destructive downward cycle, mastery experiences generate a constructive upward cycle. To increase the frequency, intensity, and quality of their clients' mastery experiences, masterful coaches discern where clients are in the TTM stages of change and then guide them to structure stage-appropriate, incremental goals that are both engaging and manageable.

The MI principle of "planning" calls for realistic, well thought-out plans that consider barriers and challenges. To strengthen goal commitment and the possibility for mastery, the coach and client collaborate to:

1.  Dream to envision the desired future
2.  Explore the client's intention with motivation and meaning

3. Create specific, measurable, and meaningful action steps
4. Examine the client's level of confidence and adjust the action steps as necessary to increase confidence
5. Create contingency plans
6. Imagine success and its positive consequences
7. Affirm commitment, strengths, and ability

As Csikszentmihalyi (2003) observes, biting off either too much or too little undermines self-efficacy because doing so generates either anxiety or boredom; this is where the research studying flow and self-efficacy converge. People with high self-efficacy experience flow more often than do people with low self-efficacy, because people with high self-efficacy know how to set goals and design projects that are just within reach.

Masterful coaches help clients transform their experiences in goal implementation into learning. Assisting clients in approaching their lives as science experiments or living laboratories can free clients to try new things and bounce back quickly from apparent setbacks. There are no failures in science, only learning experiences. Science is a "win-learn" rather than a "win-lose" enterprise. Data are collected and theories are revised until things work and fit together; this is also true when it comes to mastery experiences. If something doesn't work, we use that data to design new experiments until we find something that does work.

As in AI, coaches come from the perspective that we can always find things that work. It is important for coaches to assist clients in finding things that are important, interesting, enjoyable, and stage-appropriate from the vantage point of the client. There is little value in conducting an experiment for its own sake. It is ideally related to a larger, positive vision of who clients are, what they value, and where they want to go. It must also be grounded in the reality of what clients know and have accomplished in the past. Masterful coaches enable their clients to frame their goals and projects in these terms. They are masters of meaning-making, learning, and the pleasures in change.

## References

Bandura, A. (1986). *Social foundations of thought and action: A social cognitive theory.* Upper Saddle River, NJ: Prentice Hall.

Bandura, A. (1994). Self-efficacy. In V. S. Ramachaudran (Ed.), *Encyclopedia of human behavior* (Vol. 4, pp. 71–81). New York: Academic Press. (Reprinted in H. Friedman [Ed.], *Encyclopedia of mental health.* San Diego: Academic Press, 1998.)

Bandura, A. (1997). *Self-efficacy: The exercise of control.* Gordonsville, VA: W. H. Freeman.

Botelho, R. (2004). *Motivate healthy habits: Stepping stones to lasting change.* Rochester, NY: MHH Publications.

Boyle, P. A., Buchman, A. S., Wilson, R. S., Yu, L., Schneider, J. A., & Bennett, D. A. (2012). Effect of purpose in life on the relation between Alzheimer disease pathologic changes on cognitive function in advanced age. *Archives of General Psychiatry, 69*(5), 499–505.

Csikszentmihalyi, M. (2003). *Good business: Leadership, flow, and the making of meaning.* New York: Penguin Books.

Deci, E. (2013). *How do we both support autonomy and build accountability? A presentation for the American Journal of Health Promotion.* Retrieved April 27, 2015 from http://healthpromotionjournal.com/index.php?com _route=view_video&vid=109&close=true

Deci, E. D., & Ryan, R. M. (2002). *Handbook of self-determination research.* New York: University of Rochester Press.

Deutschman, A. (2007). *Change or die: The three keys to change at work and in life.* New York: HarperCollins.

Frankl, V. (2006). *Man's search for meaning.* Boston, MA: Beacon Press.

Humphrey, H. (2000). *Empathetic listening.* In Empathy Magic Home Page. Retrieved October 16, 2008 from http://empathymagic.com/articles/Empathic%20 Listening%20'0061.pdf

Miller, W., & Rollnick, S. (2012). *Motivational interviewing: Helping people change.* New York: Guilford Press.

Oettingen, G., & Gollwitzer, P. M. (2010). Strategies of setting and implementing goals: Mental contrasting and implementing intentions. In J. E. Maddux & J. P. Tangney (Eds.), *Social psychological foundations of clinical psychology* (pp. 114–135). New York: Guilford Press. Retrieved from http://www.psych.nyu.edu /gollwitzer/OettingenGollwitzer.pdf

Ornish, D. (2002). Statins and the soul of medicine. *The American Journal of Cardiology, 89,* 1286–1290.

Pantalon, M. V., Sledge, W. H., Bauer, S. F., Brodsky, B., Giannandrea, S., Kay, J., ... Rockland, L. (2013). Important medical decisions: Using brief motivational interviewing to enhance patients' autonomous decision-making. *Journal of Psychiatric Practice, 19*(2), 98–108.

Rosenberg, M. S. (2005). *Nonviolent communication: A language of life.* Encinitas, CA: PuddleDancer Press.

Wong, P. (1987). Meaning and purpose in life and well-being: A life span perspective. *Journal of Gerontology, 42*(1), 44–49.

# CHAPTER 7

# Readiness to Change

> *"Growth is not steady, forward, upward progression. It is instead a switchback trail; three steps forward, two back, one around the bushes, and a few simply standing, before another forward leap."*
>
> —DOROTHY CORKVILLE BRIGGS

## OBJECTIVES

After reading this chapter, you will be able to:

- Describe the transtheoretical model (TTM)
- Define the five stages of change
- Describe coaching competencies for each stage of change
- Define operant conditioning and decisional balance
- Describe the Mount Lasting Change model

## Introduction to Change of Mindset and Behavior

A primary goal of coaching is to facilitate a client's self-determined change, growth, and performance. In the health and wellness arenas, coaches and clients are particularly concerned with mindset and behavioral changes that support a higher level of health and well-being.

Fortunately, there are excellent theories and extensive research on the preconditions and processes of cognitive and behavioral change to support a coach's toolbox. One of the most important is the TTM from the field of behavioral psychology, which contributes a wealth of principles, skills, and processes to the foundation of health and wellness coaching. The TTM-inspired Mount Lasting Change pyramid described in later discussion lays out key cognitive, behavioral, and relational processes of change as a coaching framework.

## Transtheoretical Model of Change

The TTM of behavior change developed by Dr. James Prochaska and collaborators is based on decades of research evaluating and measuring behavior change for a wide variety of health behaviors, including smoking cessation, exercise adoption, and mammogram engagement. This model is a blueprint for effecting self-change in health behaviors and can be readily applied in health and wellness coaching as well as other coaching domains (Prochaska, Norcross, & DiClemente, 1994).

The TTM provides coaches with an understanding of how and when new behaviors can be adopted and sustained and why clients may struggle, fail, or quit.

Clients may decide to employ a coach because they already recognize they need and want to initiate and sustain new health- and wellness-related behaviors and they are committed to doing so. Health and wellness behavior change is particularly challenging today in light of life's heavy demands and stresses that can deplete resources for change. If it were easy, clients probably would not seek the support of a coach or they would have already made and sustained the changes they need and want.

Research has shown that self-change is a staged process in which one moves from not thinking about changing a behavior to thinking about it planning for the change and before actually starting the new behavior.

Using techniques that prematurely encourage new behaviors can discourage change. For example, people who have not yet made up their minds to change are typically not sufficiently ready to start engaging in the new behavior. Applying pressure to move them into setting goals and starting new behaviors too early can cause them to resist or withdraw from the change process.

To avoid such a setback, it is valuable to help clients consider the stage of change for each domain, and even subdomain, of health and wellness at the outset of a coaching partnership. Clients will typically be in different stages of change for different areas and also for different behaviors. They might be ready to adopt a healthy breakfast but not ready to eat more vegetables with dinner. They might be ready to walk but not participate in strength-training. They might be interested in practicing a self-compassion exercise but not in meditation. Globally, they may be more interested in dealing with stress, nutrition, or exercise first.

Once aware of the stage in which a client is for a behavior or domain, a coach can apply techniques for facilitating change that are specific and effective for that stage. Application of specific techniques at each stage may support clients in reaching their health and wellness goals more quickly and effectively as well as create a solid foundation for sustaining them.

# Stages of Change and Effective Coaching Skills for Each

Prochaska and colleagues (1994) taught that the stages through which people move are predictable and identifiable. They begin with the precontemplation stage during which they are not yet thinking about making change, all the way through to the maintenance stage where changes have been adopted as a way of life and are stable. The characteristics people exhibit at each stage are distinct and recognizable.

The five stages of change are:

1. Precontemplation (not ready for change)
2. Contemplation (thinking about change)
3. Preparation (preparing for action)
4. Action (taking action)
5. Maintenance (maintaining a positive behavior)

It is important to note that a client is not a stage but rather a client is in a particular stage related to a particular behavior or domain of change such as nutrition or physical activity.

## Precontemplation: "I Won't" or "I Can't"

When someone is not yet thinking about adopting a positive or healthy behavior, it's usually because they fall into one of two categories of the precontemplation stage; these are the clients who say "I won't" or "I can't." Those who say "I won't" are not interested in changing because they do not believe that they have a problem. Family and friends may feel otherwise and may be nagging them about it, but clients themselves fail or refuse to acknowledge a need to change, or perhaps more accurately, they may resist being changed by others. Those who say "I can't" would like to change, but they don't believe it's possible. For different reasons, both kinds of clients are not even contemplating let alone working on making a change in a particular area. Clients in the "I won't" category need to hear messages that communicate an understanding of their stage of readiness and an appreciation of their full autonomy and control over their choices. It is important that they are not made to feel judged or inadequate. Coaches should validate, with sincerity, the good reasons for the unhealthy behaviors, the needs these behaviors meet, and how they help clients cope with the demands of their lives.

Clients in the "I can't" category are aware that there are issues to be addressed and there is a need to change, but they believe change is too complicated or difficult. They may have tried and failed over and over in the past. These people may be acutely aware of their barriers and need help to look at the barriers in a positive and possibility-minded way so that they can learn from them rather than being overwhelmed by the negative emotions and low confidence generated by past failures or large roadblocks today.

Most clients will be in the contemplation and/ or preparation stage for at least one area (fitness, weight, nutrition, stress, mental, or physical health), and coaching can support them in reaching the maintenance phase (sustaining one or more new behaviors consistently week to week) within three to six months. Many clients are dealing with significant life stressors that are depleting their abilities to change, and these may be areas suited to a coaching partnership before addressing health behaviors. A coach may also be able to support a client in moving forward later in areas where they are in precontemplation when openings emerge in coaching sessions. Also, when clients progress in one area, their confidence in self-change grows and they may become ready to move forward in another area where their previous readiness was minimal.

To move forward, a client in the precontemplation stage first needs to experience genuine empathy and unconditional acceptance. This is the time to use reflections to demonstrate understanding and respect for a client's emotions and needs. A coach's ability to recognize and accept that a client does not intend to change a particular behavior is the key to building trust and future possibilities. A coach steps on a client's autonomy by encouraging him or her to move forward in making a behavior change when he or she is not ready to do so. Instead, focusing on understanding a client at a deeper level without judgment or fear supports a client's self-determination.

## COACHING CASE

**Coach Carl:** "Hello Wendy, my name is Coach Carl. I'm calling on behalf of your employer from Incredible Insurance, Inc. When you completed a health assessment last month, we noticed that you indicated that you are smoking several packs of cigarettes each day. I wondered if we could talk about ways to support you in stopping smoking."

**Wendy Well:** "Oh, yes, I figured that someone would call me. Smokers are like second-class citizens these days, you know. I suppose you are telling me I have to stop smoking, or I'll lose my insurance or get a penalty."

**Coach Carl:** "It sounds like it's been unpleasant and frustrating for you to feel as though you are being treated like a second-class citizen because you smoke."

**Wendy Well:** "Yes, it sure is. I feel like I have to hide and be embarrassed about it. I hate the critical looks I get."

**Coach Carl:** "I can imagine that you wish people would be more accepting of your need and desire to smoke."

**Wendy Well:** "Exactly. I wish they would just leave me alone and let me smoke in peace. It's the only thing that keeps me sane in my crazy life, and I don't know how I would cope without smoking."

**Coach Carl:** "I can understand how smoking is helping you cope with a lot of stress. Smokers are the only people left who take five-minute breaks and breathe deeply [said with a smile]. I'm hearing that you aren't ready right now to talk about strategies to reduce or quit smoking."

**Wendy Well:** "Yes, you've got it. I wish others would get it. Maybe someday I'll think about quitting smoking but not now."

**Coach Carl:** "I really appreciate that smoking is helping you right now. Is there another change you are ready to make that I could help you with?"

*(continued on page 97)*

With a coach, clients can sort their barriers into those that are real, feel large, and need to be put to the side right now; those that are excuses and can be reframed in new, positive ways; and those that can be overcome by tapping into the energy of deep autonomous motivation. Taking large barriers off the table in the immediate term can lower a client's resistance level to discussing any change; time may have to elapse before clients can perceive these barriers as manageable. A client doesn't have to convince a coach that the barrier feels insurmountable. This acceptance shows your clients that you are on their side. When clients are readier to work with you, find a strong positive source of self-motivation and identify other behaviors they are ready to change. When clients connect to something they really want, such as being a role model for their children by not smoking, they are far more motivated to work on other healthy changes in addition to smoking. For example, other healthy changes may include a walking program, yoga for relaxation, more fruits and vegetables, or getting in control of a large life stressor such as caring for an ill family member.

## Contemplation: "I May"

Another term for the contemplation stage is the "I may" stage. At this stage, clients are thinking about changing unhealthy behaviors or adopting healthy behaviors and are considering taking action within the next six months. They are more aware of the benefits inherent in changing and are less satisfied with their present health and well-being than are those in precontemplation around a specific behavior but still feel a sense of doubt and will delay the change.

Clients may express a fair amount of ambivalence about change, feeling that change will be difficult or even impossible to achieve. People often remain in the contemplation stage for a long time, and could be considered chronic contemplators, because they cannot imagine themselves behaving differently and/or they do not know how to change. They are still weighing the benefits of change against the effort it will take, and the balance is pretty even between the reasons to change and the reasons to stay the same. It is not until the reasons for making

the changes (the "pros") have more weight than the reasons for staying the same (the "cons") that a client becomes ready to change.

When openings emerge, those who are thinking "I may" might be willing to explore their best experiences with change in the past as well as the positive reasons for behaving in a particular way in the future. By focusing on their past accomplishments, values, and vision, they may come to appreciate how change would improve their lives. Assist these clients in connecting the dots between the changes they seek and the values and hopes for the future that they hold. Setting behavior change in this larger context makes the change more meaningful and significant. If clients have not sufficiently identified their personally compelling motivators to change, including new supportive relationships and new reasons to change, a coach can support them in thinking this through. A clear vision of what they want (not just what they don't want) is essential.

These clients need to examine not only the upside but also the downside of giving up old behaviors for new healthier behaviors. Identify which barriers are immovable for now and which can be navigated. Normalize, don't catastrophize. Most everyone is stuck in at least one life domain. Support contemplating clients in identifying and accomplishing small, realistic investigating and thinking goals at first to enhance motivation and/or confidence, thereby empowering them to be more confident in their ability to change.

Clients can move beyond the contemplation stage by connecting to their strengths and getting excited about the possibilities that would emerge with change. The discovery work alone may be enough to move them to the next stage of change. Increasing their awareness of compelling reasons to change and getting them to connect with people who have successfully made similar changes are key change strategies.

When appropriate, coaches can ask whether clients want them to share important scientific facts about the benefits of a behavior. Coaches can assist clients with discovering and sorting through the benefits for change, and these can become positive and even powerful motivators.

In the contemplation stage, stage-appropriate goals include mindset shifts through reading, thinking, talking, listening, discovering, and deciding—often not actually doing the particular behavior. Or sometimes, a client might also adopt the Nike "just do it" mantra and take tiny behavioral steps like five-minute walks, 10 minutes of yoga poses, or an apple a day while sorting through ambivalence. A series of small successes without a larger commitment can also build self-efficacy and improve readiness.

## COACHING CASE Continued

**Wendy Well:** "So you really aren't going to try to press me to stop smoking?"

**Coach Carl:** "I'm really not. Whether you do or don't is completely your choice. I'm here to support you when you are ready to start thinking about it and perhaps help you make a different change that seems more manageable."

**Wendy Well:** "Well, I'm not interested in giving up cigarettes; they help me calm down during my stressful work days."

**Coach Carl:** "I appreciate that smoking helps you get through your stressful days."

**Wendy Well:** "I have been working overtime for months on an urgent project, barely getting downtime at home let alone exercise—nothing healthy, really."

**Coach Carl:** "This is a tough phase with no time to take care of yourself. And you don't have time to exercise."

**Wendy Well:** "I've never been someone who exercises."

**Coach Carl:** "So exercising seems like a stretch."

**Wendy Well:** "Maybe not. I was just thinking that if I could walk on the treadmill or something, I might feel a little less stressed out. Could be a good anxiety reliever, but I don't know. Like I said, I've never exercised before."

## Preparation: "I Will"

The preparation stage is also known as the "I will" stage. In the preparation stage, ambivalent feelings have been largely overcome. Clients have strengthened their motivation, and they are planning to take some action within the next month. These clients have one or more strong motivators. They know what their barriers are, and they have come up with some possible solutions that provide some hope for success. If these thinking tasks, developing strategies to navigate barriers, are not accomplished, then clients will likely remain in the contemplation stage.

During preparation, clients experiment with their possible solutions, discard the ones that do not

## COACHING CASE Continued

**Coach Carl:** "Tell me more about the appeal of exercise."

**Wendy Well:** "My husband started to run about nine months ago, and I've been amazed at how much it has changed his body and his attitude. I've been a little envious. Plus, I've noticed that after sitting all day at the office, I just don't feel good."

**Coach Carl:** "You think exercising could improve your attitude and help you feel better after a long day of being sedentary. What are some possibilities for adding exercise?"

**Wendy Well:** "I thought about the treadmill but realized it is spring and I'd rather be outside. There is a nice park just a block from work, but honestly, I don't think I would ever go during the workday. So I've been thinking about walking when my husband starts his run."

**Coach Carl:** "Sounds as though you've thought through a few options that won't work and have one in mind that could. What do you like about the idea of walking while he runs?"

**Wendy Well:** "He would inspire me to get moving. And he would be glad that he is helping me because he worries about my smoking."

work, and think up new approaches. In this stage, a coach can support clients in solidifying plans for change. For example, a client could write down a formal statement of what they are committing themselves to do, containing specific details of what, when, and how. Additionally with a coach, a client could brainstorm to identify the many small steps that could be taken as long as they are realistic.

If clients exhibit ambivalence, resistance, or fear of failure, it is important to explore the challenges and identify new ways to navigate around their challenges. However, a coach must be cautious not to add to the resistance by telling a client what to do. Honor a client's competence, and fears, by asking the client to take the lead in co-creating solutions and strategies.

Discuss situations clients think could be problematic when they actually start the behavior and have them develop multiple possible strategies before they begin.

## Action: "I Am"

During the next stage, which lasts six months or longer, clients are working on building new relationships, practicing new behaviors, and establishing new habits. The action stage is also known as the "I am" stage.

Here, clients may have to concentrate hard while practicing fledgling new behaviors and refining their lifestyles. In this stage, clients have identified one or more new behaviors they want to establish and are doing them consistently, building up week by week, month by month, to a target level. For example, a client may be working toward more cardiovascular exercise, for instance, three to four times a week for 15–60 minutes at a time at a moderate to high level of intensity, or he or she may be meeting a specific set of nutrition criteria he or she has agreed on with a physician. A client may also be striving toward a goal that will provide some relief from a life overflowing with stress.

When clients are in the "I am" stage for a particular behavior, it is important that they keep their strengths and values at the top of their minds to get on and stay on track. It's also valuable for them to engage social connections or develop new relationships with people who share their interests and behavioral goals. The more modes of support they can identify, the better.

## COACHING CASE Continued

(One month later)

**Coach Carl:** "It's been a month since we last spoke. I've missed connecting with you. Tell me what is going well with the goals that you set for yourself in our last session."

**Wendy Well:** "I'm glad we are reconnecting too. I think I am off to a pretty good start! For the last three weeks, I have walked at least two days each week for about an hour each time."

**Coach Carl:** "Wow! That is a great start! When we set the goal, you were aiming for 30 minutes, and you've been walking for an hour. What helped you go beyond your original goal?"

**Wendy Well:** "First, I find that my husband and I are in much better moods in the evenings after we have both exercised. We laugh more in the evening. And remember that I told you work was stressful? That hasn't changed, but I feel like the walking helps me destress and let go of it for the evening."

**Coach Carl:** "That's great to hear. What strengths and strategies have you used to be so consistent in walking?"

**Wendy Well:** "I have gotten in the habit of not planning to run any errands until after my walk on those days. I also just try to remember how good the walk felt the time before."

**Coach Carl:** "Congratulations on your progress and perseverance! With cold winter days coming, I wonder what you are thinking it will take to stay on track."

Through gradual changes and small achievable steps, clients can feel successful early. It's important to anticipate situations that could be problematic and encourage clients to develop multiple possible strategies to handle these situations before they come up.

Coaches should anticipate and be prepared for lapses in behavior and support clients in reframing lapses as temporary setbacks. These incidents are best perceived as important learning opportunities rather than failures. An all-or-nothing mentality about goals can lead to guilt, self-blame, and reasons to quit. A client could even benefit from conducting a safe, planned lapse, such as a day without exercise or a meal during which he or she can eat anything, to develop new mental skills, perspective, and resilience under a controlled situation.

Because there is a high risk of a return to the preparation stage, discussions to process the learning from setbacks and reframe them as sources of valuable learning are important. A client may lapse once in his or her execution of a desired behavior or may cease to engage in the desired behaviors all together for a week or more. These situations provide an opportunity to explore a client's response to the situation, the perceived loss of control, and the help or hindrance of social connections. A coach can support clients in exploring their challenging situations and to learn from them for the future. Assisting clients in developing new relationships with people who share their interests and behavioral goals can make significant differences. With the right modeling and supportive environment, clients will be more likely to make progress in the action stage of change.

## Maintenance: "I Still Am"

When a client is in the maintenance stage for a behavior, s/he is in the "I still am" stage. This stage begins when the new behavior change has become a habit and is done automatically—usually at least six months after the initial behavior has changed. Clients are now confident that they can maintain the new behavior, and they would rate their confidence to maintain the new behavior at a level of 8 or 9 out of 10. In this stage, their self-efficacy is both high and self-reinforcing.

Just because clients progress to the maintenance level does not mean they don't need to continue working diligently to maintain a new behavior and prevent relapse. (Nor does it necessarily mean that they will no longer need or want a coach.) There are different sets of risks in maintenance, including boredom and the danger of gradually slipping back into old, less healthful habits.

Lapses, in which people temporarily abandon new behaviors, can occur during the maintenance period just as easily as it can during the action stage. If and when this happens, clients often need assistance to set new goals and get refocused. For example, they may benefit from signing up for an event related to the goal, taking up a new type of exercise, trying a new but related skill, or helping others who are just getting started. This can be easier in maintenance than in action because the clients have already come to experience the value and benefits of their new behavioral patterns. Lapses in this stage don't usually produce any significant alteration in the health and fitness benefits of the behavior change, which means people can more easily and quickly get back on track. Learning to make such adjustments is indeed a sign of being in the maintenance stage of change.

Relapses can be more challenging in any stage of change. As extended abandonments of new behaviors, relapses lead to the reduction or even to the disappearance of benefits. To reverse a relapse, it is important to revisit, revise, and reconnect clients with their strengths, values, resources, visions, goals, and motivators. In addition to exploring lessons learned, it is important to go back and restart the preparation and action process with judgment-free listening, inquiries, and reflections. The more vividly clients can remember and reconnect with their capacity to put their strengths to work, the more they will develop the self-efficacy and regain their sense of control.

The five stages of change are illustrated in Figure 7.1; you can see that lapses and relapses are a normal part of the change process.

**Figure 7.1.** Stages of change.

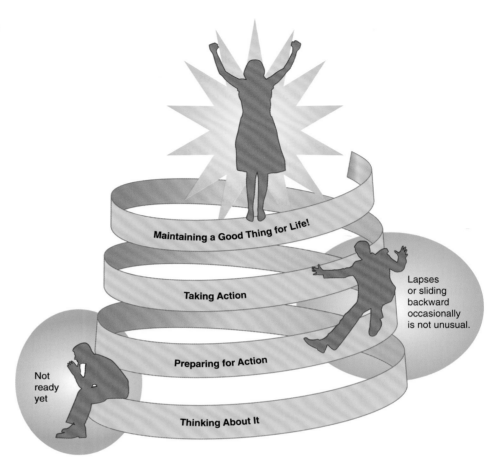

Table 7.1 provides a summary of the coaching skills that are useful for each stage of change with reference to the International Coach Federation's Core Coaching Competencies (International Coach Federation [ICF], 2015).

## Processes of Change

Prochaska recognized that some people were ready to change and others were not and that different strategies had to be used for people in different stages of readiness. After surveying a wide variety of different psychotherapeutic models, Prochaska and his collaborators (1994) put together the TTM to identify what processes worked best for people in different stages of change. With Carlo DiClemente, 10 such processes that describe what people actually do to change were identified. Five are cogni-

tive processes and five are behavioral processes of change.

Cognitive processes encompass a wide range of reflective learning processes in which people are sorting out their thoughts, feelings, and desires regarding a particular health-promoting change. These processes, which often take place over a period of several months or even years, include:

1. Getting information: finding out about all the benefits (e.g., medical and life) of doing a behavior
2. Being moved emotionally: taking to heart the health and life benefits of a behavior and using these benefits to ignite a client's drive to change
3. Considering how one's behavior affects others: for example, thinking one's children may be learning from witnessing a parent's positive behavior

| Table 7.1 | Coaching Skills for Behavior Change | |
|---|---|---|
| **Stage** | **Skills to Use** | **Explanation** |
| **Precontemplation: I won't** | Listening<br>Compassion<br>Mindfulness<br>Inquiry<br>Reflections<br>Autonomy<br>Reframing<br>Sharing<br>Brainstorming<br>AI and MI | We've all been there, and the client needs to know we understand their needs, emotions, and circumstances. This is not the time to judge but to empathize. Compassion, "to suffer with," is the operative word. Accepting people right where they are without lecturing them about where they ought to be will build the trust and intimacy so necessary to being a catalyst for change. (See ICF Core Competencies 3 and 4.)<br><br>The *I won'ts* need to bolster their appreciation of the pros. |
| **I can't** | Listening<br>Compassion<br>Mindfulness<br>Inquiry<br>Reflections<br>Affirmation<br>Reframing<br>Sharing<br>Self-efficacy<br>Sorting barriers<br>AI and MI | *I can'ts* need to bolster their confidence for overcoming the cons. We can also offer to help them sort through their barriers.<br><br>Everyone in precontemplation needs not only reasons why but also hope when it comes to the prospects for change. |
| **Contemplation: I may** | Listening<br>Compassion<br>Mindfulness<br>Inquiry<br>Reflections<br>Affirmation<br>Reframing<br>Sharing<br>Brainstorming<br>AI and MI<br>Self-efficacy | Contemplators need to get in touch and stay connected with their strengths, core values, and autonomous motivation for change. Identifying strengths, values, and motivators will assist contemplators in completing the vision of the coaching process, giving them more clarity on where they want to go and why.<br><br>Contemplators need to find strong motivators. They need to identify their barriers and come up with possible solutions. Accomplishing these three thinking tasks moves contemplators forward into preparation. Sharing information as well as stories related to the possibilities for and benefits of making a change can make an invaluable contribution to the client's change process. (See ICF Core Competencies 7 and 8.) |
| **Preparation: I will** | Listening<br>Compassion<br>Inquiry<br>Reflections<br>Affirmation<br>AI<br>Brainstorming<br>Experimenting<br>Committing<br>Testing<br>Scheduling<br>Accountability | Once people have strong motivators, know their barriers, and have thought of some possible solutions, it's time for the coach to work with them on designing actions (ICF Core Competencies 9 and 10). This starts with exploring their positive core (AI, Chapter 4) through powerful questioning (ICF Core Competency 6). Although we may want to teach them the tricks to being successful, it's better to assist them in discovering, designing, committing to, and experimenting with their own strategies for success. Those are the ones that are more likely to stick. |

*(continued on next page)*

| Table 7.1 | Coaching Skills for Behavior Change (Continued) | |
|---|---|---|
| **Stage** | **Skills to Use** | **Explanation** |
| **Action: I am** | **Listening** **Inquiry** **Reflections** **Support** **Self-efficacy** **Normalizing** **Calibrating** **Reengineering** **Environmental** **Design** | If ever there were a time for a coach to be a cheerleader and a champion, it's in the action stage of change. The client has started on the path—he or she needs our confidence, energy, and commitment to believe he or she can stay on the path (ICF Core Competency 9). We walk a tightrope here between support and challenge. Clients need to be inspired. Too much support, and we baby them; too much challenge, and we overwhelm them. To inspire them, we keep just the right amount of tension on the line. As clients run into challenging situations, the coach helps them analyze them and come up with relapse prevention plans. |
| **Maintenance: I still am** | **Listening** **Inquiry** **Reflections** **Support** **Inspiration** **Modeling** **Improvisation** **Creativity** **Autonomous** **   motivation** | If it takes 21 days to develop a new, easy habit, it may take 21 months to develop a new lifestyle. During the process, clients will discover new and exciting things about themselves; they will also encounter challenges and setbacks as well as boredom and discouragement. Helping clients develop into role models for others is a powerful way for them to stay motivated. By being flexible, creative, and inventive, coaches can assist clients in staying engaged. This is part and parcel of managing progress and accountability (ICF Core Competency 11), which may be too heavy for some clients to handle without continued experimentation and improvisation (ICF Core Competency 9). |

AI, appreciative inquiry; MI, motivational interviewing.

4. Self-image: connecting the dots and seeking congruence between one's vision, values, and behaviors to enhance integrity

5. Social norms: connecting and talking with like-minded people who are all working on the same behavior (e.g., a support or special interest group)

Behavioral processes encompass a wide range of action-oriented learning processes in which people are experimenting with new health-promoting behaviors and adopting the ones that work. These processes include:

1. Making a commitment: for example, writing down exactly what new behavior will be done and when

2. Using cues: for example, designing environmental reminders to do what is planned

3. Using substitution: replacing an old health-risk behavior with a new health-promoting behavior (e.g., substituting carrot sticks or a straw for a cigarette)

4. Social support: recruiting family and friends to help with behavior change by asking for specific forms of support; this requires clients to think carefully about what they would like someone to do and then to ask the person on their support team to do it

5. Rewards: setting up reward systems for having completed action goals

## Supporting Clients in Moving Through the Stages of Change

After establishing trust and rapport with an orientation around the clients' strengths and values, it is valuable to encourage clients to identify what stages of readiness they believe they are in with regard to their potential areas of focus or any life issues related to their health and well-being. This alone can generate engaging conversations as to why they picked the stage they picked, what got them to where they are, and what goals or behaviors they want to focus on first in moving forward. This also supports in developing a client's sense of competence and autonomy in moving toward change.

## Supporting Self-Efficacy

One goal of using the TTM process is to increase a client's sense of self-efficacy or belief that one has the capability to make a change in a desired area. Self-efficacy describes the circular relationship between belief and action; the more you believe you can do something, the more likely you are to do it. The more you do something successfully, the more you believe that you will be able to do it again.

The opposite is also true; the more you believe that you cannot do something, the less likely you are to do it. The more you do something unsuccessfully, the less you believe that you will be able to do it again. In other words, to quote an old adage, "Nothing succeeds like success." Therefore, it is important that clients set appropriate goals—ones that correspond to a client's stage of change and capability. The potential consequence of inappropriate goals is that the client may lapse, possibly setting up a series of relapses. That's also why it is so important to correctly determine a client's stage or readiness to change (e.g., whether you are working with an "I may" or an "I will" person). In other words, it can be risky for a client in the contemplation stage for a behavior to set late-stage behavioral goals. Instead, a more appropriate goal type would be a thinking goal, which encourages the exploration of motivators and challenges.

When clients have experienced a challenging situation and have had a lapse, the coach can work to reframe the experience as a learning experience.

## COACHING CASE

**Wendy Well:** "I really failed at my goal to not smoke over the weekend."

**Coach Carl:** "I know that was a challenge for you, and I hear your disappointment."

**Wendy Well:** "Frustrated, mad at myself. I know I can do better than this."

**Coach Carl:** "If you want to reach this goal, I know you can. Let's rewind and see what can be learned here. What factors do you think contributed to your decision to smoke after you had committed to not smoking on the weekend?"

**Wendy Well:** "I know exactly what happened. I was out running errands, so I was in my car all day, and I didn't stop to eat lunch. Before I knew it, I was smoking in my car."

**Coach Carl:** "Connect the dots for me. How did that situation lead to smoking?"

**Wendy Well:** "First, once I was hungry, I had no willpower. And I wanted something to put in my mouth."

**Coach Carl:** "Interesting, there may be something here to learn about your triggers."

**Wendy Well:** "Yes, I'm definitely less likely to make a good choice when I'm hungry."

**Coach Carl:** "Interesting observation. How will you apply this learning in the future?"

## Operant Conditioning

Another way to engage clients in the processes of change, especially in the behavioral processes, is to focus on the relationship of a behavior and its consequences. Known as operant conditioning, or learning through positive and negative reinforcement, it is a form of learning that takes place when an instance of spontaneous behavior is either reinforced or discouraged by its consequences.

Successful operant conditioning looks for the antecedent conditions that may trigger an undesired behavior. For example, missing breakfast may lead to overeating at lunch, which may lead to feelings of guilt, which may lead to irritability. This irritability may lead to abandonment of any improved eating habits for that day. The end result can be an ice cream binge after dinner. When a behavior chain is identified, assisting clients to alter a behavior earlier in the chain instead of later can generate significant shifts and benefits.

It is often easier to manipulate the antecedents than to modify the consequences or behaviors. Examples of antecedent conditions could include a long drive to get to the gym, an unpleasant workout environment, driving by a favorite ice cream shop, a particularly stressful day, or negative self-talk. For example, stressful workdays and self-statements, such as "I am overwhelmed and can't deal with everything," may lead to overeating at dinner on a continual basis. It may be helpful to create a goal that helps clients relieve some of the stress during the day or before eating in addition to their goals that relate to eating.

## Readiness to Change Assessment

The following readiness to change assessment (Table 7.2) can be used with clients to prioritize the behaviors they want to change and rate their confidence in their ability to change.

It's not important that clients use the formal names of the stages themselves. It may be better to simply have clients choose the descriptive statement that best describes where they are with respect to changing a particular behavior:

- I won't do it.
- I can't do it.
- I may do it.
- I will do it.
- I am doing it.
- I am still doing it.

Once a client has become familiar with the stages of change, a coaching session may flow according to the following pattern:

- Explore the client's strengths, core values, and primary motivators or reasons for change.
- Co-identify the client's stage of change and one or more appropriate cognitive or behavioral goals.
- Co-design strategies that will promote quick wins and self-efficacy with those cognitive or behavioral goals.

- Discuss challenges, as appropriate, that may interfere with behavior change and stimulate generative thought about possible solutions.
- Elicit the client's commitments as to the steps he or she will take and the efforts he or she will make in the week ahead.
- Reconfirm the client's readiness to change and willingness to move forward.

## Decisional Balance

An effective way to engage clients in the processes of change, especially the cognitive processes, is to encourage them to weigh the pros and cons of a particular behavior or behavioral change. Known as a decisional balance (Janis & Mann, 1977), such weighing increases the chance of successful behavior change by taking into consideration:

- The pros or gains for self, gains for others, approval of others, and self-approval
- The cons or losses for self, losses for others, disapproval of others, and self-disapproval

## COACHING CASE

**Wendy Well:** "I want to stop smoking for my health, so I won't get sick down the road."

**Coach Carl:** "Tell me more about what you imagine is possible for you 'down the road' that isn't now."

**Wendy Well:** "I have three grandchildren whom I really love and with whom I want to be able to spend time."

**Coach Carl:** "One of the most important reasons for you to make a change is to be able to enjoy time with your grandchildren."

**Wendy Well:** "Yes. Another reason is that I really want to stop smoking now because my children will not allow my grandchildren to come into my house because I smoke, and I want to be able to bake cookies and play games with my grandchildren."

| **Table 7.2** | **Readiness to Change Assessment** |
| --- | --- |

Research has shown that self-change is a staged process. We move from not thinking about changing a behavior to thinking about it, to planning to change, and then to testing out ways to do it before we actually start. When thinking about changing or adopting a behavior, ask yourself the following:

1. Why do I really want to change the behavior; what makes the change important to me (the benefits or pros)?
2. Why shouldn't I try to change the behavior; what is in my way (the obstacles or cons)?
3. Do my pros outweigh my cons?
4. What would it take for me to change the behavior and overcome my cons? What's my strategy?
5. Can I really do it?

To move forward, it is best if you believe in your ability to change; the pros outweigh the cons and you have realistic strategies to overcome the cons. Behavioral scientists recognize five stages of readiness to change a behavior:

1. Precontemplation ("I won't or I can't in the next six months.")
2. Contemplation ("I may in the next six months.")
3. Preparation ("I will in the next month.")
4. Action ("I'm doing it now.")
5. Maintenance ("I've been doing it for at least six months.")

A number of techniques can help you move from not thinking to thinking, to planning, to doing, and to continue doing. Determining how ready you are to change a behavior can assist your coach in helping you make that change. The following questions can assist you and your coach with making that determination. Your answers will help your coach guide the conversation so that you can move through the stages of change and reach your goals.

1. The goal or behavior I want to work on first is:
2. My reasons for wanting to accomplish this goal or change this behavior are:
3. The strengths, aptitudes, values, and resources that I can draw upon include:
4. The main challenges I will face while changing this behavior are:
5. My strategies to move forward and meet those challenges are:
6. The efforts I made toward changing this behavior in the last week are:
7. My goal for next week with respect to this behavior is:
8. My readiness to change the behavior is (circle the level that best describes where you are):
   - I won't do it.
   - I can't do it.
   - I may do it.
   - I will do it.
   - I am doing it.
   - I am still doing it.

Pros, benefits, and motivators are the good things about doing a new healthy behavior. They are what the client will get if he or she behaves in this new healthy way. Through inquiry, the coach can support the client in moving from a general, nonspecific pro to a specific, personal, positive motivator.

Cons, barriers, and challenges are things that make it hard to do a new healthy behavior. By getting clients to sort through their barriers, the coach can assist them in discovering that some barriers are large and only time will change them, whereas some can be overcome by a strong enough pro or motivator. For example, the young executive who was working 14 hours a day in his first job trying to make a name for himself had absolutely no time to exercise regularly until an attractive young woman who worked out regularly joined his firm. He then somehow found the time to go to gym because he wanted to get to know her. Some barriers can be overcome by a strong enough motivator.

Although it may seem counterintuitive, researchers have found that the pros have to outweigh the cons for someone to actually start and continue a new behavior successfully. This means it is important to help clients in the early stages of change who have not yet started to do a behavior to find personally salient, specific, positive pros or motivators while they honestly sort out their cons.

When a client is thinking about changing a behavior, a coach may use the following inquiries:

1. What is leading you to want to try and change the behavior? (What are the pros?)
2. What are the reasons you shouldn't try to change the behavior? (What are the cons?)
3. What would it take for you to change the behavior? (What's your strategy to overcome your cons?)

Cognitive processes comprise the key work for clients in the early stages of change. By assisting such clients with articulating strong, personal, specific, and positive motivators and by assisting them in discovering not only their barriers to change but also possible solutions or workarounds, coaches help clients get ready for action.

If a client is in the "I can't" stage and totally focused on barriers and all the reasons that they cannot make a change, acknowledge the value of their appreciating their barriers. If the three tasks of a person in the early stages are finding a motivator, knowing their barriers, and coming up with some possible solutions, this person has one of the three tasks completed. He or she is acutely aware of the barriers. The work of coaching is to make sure the other two tasks get done.

## The Mount Lasting Change Model

Drawing from the cognitive and behavioral processes of the TTM as well as from evidence-based principles of behavioral psychology and positive psychology and experience in coaching clients and training and testing coaches, Wellcoaches created a graphic metaphor for the coaching process: Mount Lasting Change. This behavior change pyramid provides a guide to what it takes to make lasting changes in mindset, behavior, self-awareness, and self-image (Fig. 7.2).

The base level of the pyramid represents the vision and higher purpose for change. First, the clients decide to take charge. Then, they define what it would like to be their best selves—what they value most about life and what they are striving for. It is also important to identify the skills and knowledge to reach one's "best self" as well as the strategies for using strengths to handle challenges. The next level addresses how the vision is turned into a realistic plan, including behavioral goals, one's support team, and how to increase confidence. Then a commitment is formalized. The third level depicts the doing process (specific behavioral goals) with early wins and constant fine-tuning. The fourth level represents the approach to sustaining new behaviors. The top is the "best self." This is what a client yearns to become or uncover through the change process.

Change isn't a linear process along which one proceeds from the bottom directly to the top of the pyramid. Clients cycle up and down the five levels, sometimes for years. When they don't make lasting change, they typically have missing or weak building blocks. A coach works with a client to lay down the structure and assemble the building blocks to get to lasting change and the client's best self.

The Mount Lasting Change pyramid can be applied to any area of health, well-being, and performance in life and work. One can use the pyramid for single behaviors (e.g., three 30-minute walks per week) or groups of related behaviors (e.g., nutrition including five servings of fruits and vegetables per day, balanced breakfast five days a week, and healthy snacks five days a week).

## Vision Level

The bottom "vision level" of the pyramid is the foundation for change. It is essential not to rush through this level. Devoting the time to generously exploring a client's positive core—the vision-level building blocks—prior to moving into preparation and action is enlightening and valuable. Revisiting

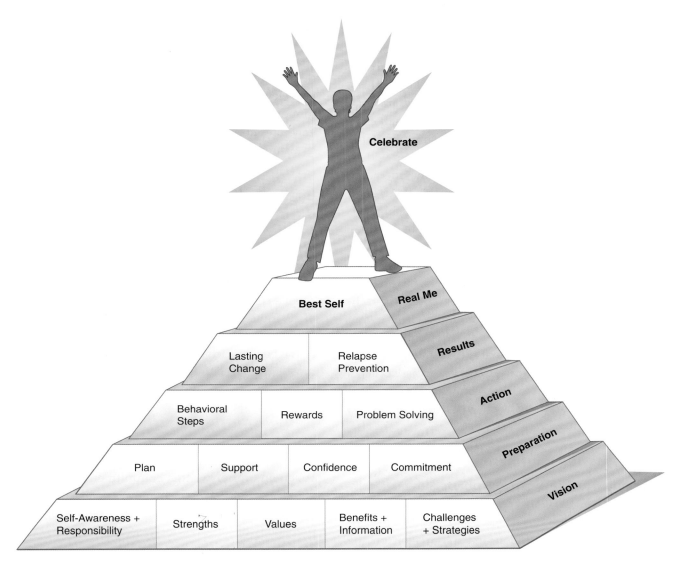

**Figure 7.2.** Mount Lasting Change.

and reinforcing the vision building blocks along the way breathes life and inspiration into the change process.

## Self-Awareness and Responsibility

Developing mindfulness and self-awareness of where the client stands with all of the building blocks is an ever-present theme. Taking charge and personal responsibility for change is the call to action, activating autonomy and self-determination.

People choose to make specific changes at specific times and for specific reasons when they are ready, willing, and able.

## Strengths

The change process is much more likely to succeed if clients identify and stay connected to the strengths and abilities that have proven successful in other parts of their lives. Building on what's working now is a key coaching approach.

## Values

This building block is at the center of the foundation because it represents both the higher purpose and deeper meaning for the change. One's values, when clearly articulated and kept in view, are what keep them going in the face of big and small challenges. What people value or treasure about the benefits of change is highly personal, ranges widely, and changes over time. Some values include being a role model, having peace of mind, looking good or youthful, living in balance, and exercising self-control. To discover client values, ask about who they want to be and why they want to be that way. Of course, one can't become that person overnight, but one can start doing the things that person would do. Acting "as if" is a great way to get on track. Coaching discussions often center around a client giving himself or herself permission to live from his or her values, especially when that means saying "no" to others to practice self-care. Coaches can assist clients in recognizing that setting boundaries to support self-care undergirds being one's best in life and work.

## Benefits and Information

One must identify, explore, prioritize, and emotionally connect with the list of potential benefits to be derived from making lasting change. When needed, providing just-in-time education and information on the new behavior(s) will be important for keeping a client interested in experimenting with new behaviors.

## Challenges and Strategies

Identifying and exploring significant challenges, such as competing priorities, lack of time, lack of confidence, and the benefits of not changing are ongoing life processes. Raising awareness of how challenges might be both harmful and helpful is important thinking/feeling work for those in the early stages of change.

The thinking/feeling work around challenges then leads to the thinking/feeling work around realistic strategies for moving forward. Some clients will get so excited about a new interest that challenges will seemingly fade from view. Other clients will want to develop specific strategies for dealing with challenges, especially if they have a long history of derailment. Either way, the key to masterful coaching is to elevate a client's confidence in his or her ability to move forward successfully. At its core, coaching generates hope in a client's ability to change as well as awareness of realistic strategies that work.

## Preparation Level

### Confidence

Before proceeding and while on the change path, it is vitally important to have a moderate to high level of confidence in one's ability to be successful. If a client's confidence level is less than a score of 7 out of 10, more work is needed to increase the level to at least a 7 or an 8. One of the most important goals of the behavior change process is self-efficacy; one must have the confidence that one has the ability to initiate and sustain a desired behavior, even in the face of challenges.

### Commitment

When an oral or written commitment is made to another person—a family member, friend, colleague, physician, or coach—to establish a new habit, the probability of success is increased.

### Support

Making changes can be tough and having support from family, friends, or colleagues, who can help us work through the change process, stay on track, and provide positive feedback, is extremely valuable. It's often helpful for clients to ask for support and be specific, explaining the kind of support that is working or not working. Clients appreciate and experience more success when they have support for their autonomously selected goals.

### Plan

The details are crucial. Developing and updating a detailed plan describing scheduling and preparation, as well as clearly defining the behavioral goal (what, when, and how), is an important activity. Tracking performance is also important—using journals or logs, for example, to record how we eat, exercise, and relax.

## Action Level

### Behavioral Steps

Choosing, refining, and committing to specific behavioral goals which are realistic while challenging is the all-important "doing" part of behavior change. Committing to the mastery of a new behavior in three months or so, and then maintaining it for a further three to six months, reaching high self-efficacy, is a good target for change. The goal should be specific and measurable; for example, replace "exercising more" with "I will walk four days a week for 30 minutes at a moderate intensity." Building up to a three-month behavioral goal should progress gradually each week in manageable steps. Some weeks, more progress will be made than others. A good starting point would be "walking four days for 10 minutes" or "walking two days for 20 minutes."

### Problem Solving

Although challenges and strategies are addressed on the vision level as part of the foundation for change, clients inevitably encounter challenges and setbacks along the way to reaching and mastering their behavioral goals. Coaches can assist clients in viewing such times in a positive light as opportunities to learn and grow. An effective problem-solving process, including brainstorming, enables rapid self-awareness, increased desire to stay on track, and prompt corrective actions, which may include brainstorming and experimenting with new action strategies or even tweaking the behavioral goals themselves. The secret is to normalize and appreciate such experiences for the gifts they have to offer rather than to fret or catastrophize and begin a downward spiral.

### Rewards

To reinforce a client's motivation and confidence, it is important to experience quick "wins," to enjoy

extrinsic rewards, and to savor the intrinsic value of behavioral changes. Clients generally start to feel better, stronger, lighter, or more energetic, for example, when they start to exercise more, eat better, relax more, be more engaged with life, or have more fun. They need to mindfully observe, enjoy, and celebrate such rewards to fully engage with and sustain the change process.

## Results Level

### Lasting Change

The diligent effort to build up to a behavioral goal and embrace the challenges along the way has a big payoff when clients are successful. The key is to move from extrinsic incentives to intrinsic motivation and contentment. That is the work of masterful coaching.

### Relapse Prevention

Even after one has mastered a new behavior, there is still potential to get sidetracked. Shift happens. New challenges emerge as environments and motivations change. Developing strategies to prevent relapses is the thinking/feeling work required when a client has reached the maintenance stage of change.

## Best Self

One of the big bonuses of lasting change is the expansion of one's sense of self. Often, one's best self is buried under extra physical and emotional weight and stress and is revealed when change has been experienced, even mastered. A coach encourages a client to take time to notice, embrace, enjoy his or her best self, and celebrate!

## General Suggestions for Coaching Change in Light of the Transtheoretical Model

Ambivalence, the existence of coexisting and conflicting feelings that create a decisional balance that doesn't lean toward pros or cons, can be a major factor inhibiting clients' commitment to change. Feeling ambivalent is a common and perfectly normal state of mind. Guide clients to accept their ambivalence rather than to fight it in order to better work their way through it. It may always be present to some extent, and that's OK. Ambivalence doesn't need to be completely resolved for clients to get started and be successful with change. For example, some people may always be ambivalent toward getting up early to exercise, but they continue anyway because the intrinsic rewards make it worth doing.

If ambivalence jeopardizes your clients' commitment, then it is a problem. If it simply makes them question their commitment, and does little more than lead to a temporary detour now and then, it can be positive experience as they develop resilience and an ability to get back on track. Self-awareness of their positive core and goal setting through lapses and relapse are powerful tools for dealing with ambivalence.

Clients may underestimate the power of a personal coaching program at the beginning. With your help, they will make changes they didn't realize were possible. As their confidence in changing grows, their readiness to change will spill over to other areas of their health and fitness and even other areas of their lives.

Change in one area of life can have a mobilizing effect on changing another area. Coaches will find that when clients have success in areas where their readiness to change is more advanced, they may progress past contemplation in the more difficult areas, powered by new self-efficacy.

Assist clients in frequently connecting with their positive core, especially their strengths, aptitudes, values, and resources for learning and growth. This will assist them in maintaining a hopeful and positive relationship to the prospect of behavior change. Remind your clients that change can be uncomfortable and difficult in the beginning. This is normal when people are stepping out of their comfort zones and seeking to make conscious changes.

Reassure clients that lapses are common during the early stages of change; that is why they will need a lot of encouragement and support when they first get started. If clients are struggling with change, the coach can reassure them that what they are experiencing is a normal part of the change process and let them know that they are doing something that is difficult for most people. It is a good time to remind them of progress they have made to date—such as hiring a coach! Most people underestimate their ability to change and lack the tools and process to facilitate change. A coach can help clients raise their level of confidence by never losing sight of their positive cores. "You CAN do it!" is a key framework of masterful coaching.

Coaches help clients develop internal motivation and focus less on external motivators by having them look inside and focus on changing behaviors for themselves and not for anyone else. If a client's motivation originates externally (i.e., "I'm doing this for my spouse/children/employer/etc."), it can wobble and then lead to guilt, frustration, anger, and often quitting. When clients can honestly say "I'm doing this because it will make me feel good and feel good about myself," then they have internal or intrinsic motivation. The guilt-inducing, self-esteem–based "I should do this" is usually counterproductive because it fosters inner criticism which is depleting. Client should focus on their internal and positive motivation and not on externally induced pressure and validation.

Common sources of ambivalence include:

- I don't really want to do this (I don't have a good enough reason).
- I can't do this.
- I have never done this.
- I don't have the time.
- I can't get started.
- It's too hard.
- I won't be able to . . . (drink beer with my friends, enjoy parties, eat what my family eats, etc.)

At the conclusion of a coaching session, a coach should consider: "Is this client really in the stage I think they are in or have they moved back into an earlier stage, and I need to help them set more thinking/feeling goals instead of behavioral goals?" When the coach is not on the same page as the client, the dynamic dialogue can disappear, leaving a sense of disconnection.

If clients have not made significant progress on chosen goals over 3–4 weeks and the goals are not unrealistic, it may be time to honestly question whether they are truly committed to those goals. They may want to change their goals or even their approach. For example, a client may benefit from a different intervention, such as a dietitian, personal trainer, or psychotherapist, or a more prescriptive or structured program with a lot of education. Often, clients receive such honest questions as a "wakeup call" that renews their commitment to change.

The breakthrough comes when clients take control and responsibility for their own well-being and health, the change process, and becoming connected with their own motivators. This will unleash their inner resources to navigate the obstacle course of change.

## References

International Coach Federation. *Core competencies.* Retrieved March 25, 2014 from http://coach federation.org/credential/landing.cfm?Item Number=2206&navItemNumber=576

Janis, I., & Mann, L. (1977). *Decision making: A psychological analysis of conflict, choice, and commitment.* New York: The Free Press.

Prochaska, J. O., Norcross, J. C., & DiClemente, C. C. (1994). *Changing for good: A revolutionary program that explains the six stages of change and teaches you how to free yourself from bad habits.* New York: HarperCollins.

## Suggested Readings

Bandura, A. (1986). *Social foundations of thought and action: A social cognitive theory.* Upper Saddle River, NJ: Prentice Hall.

Bandura, A. (1994). Self-efficacy. In V. S. Ramachaudran (Ed.), *Encyclopedia of human behavior* (Vol. 4, pp. 71–81). New York: Academic Press. (Reprinted in H. Friedman [Ed.], *Encyclopedia of mental health.* San Diego: Academic Press, 1998.)

Bandura, A. (1997). *Self-efficacy: The exercise of control.* Gordonsville, VA: W. H. Freeman.

Botelho, R. (2004). *Motivate healthy habits: Stepping stones to lasting change.* Rochester, NY: MHH Publications.

Deutschman, A. (2007). *Change or die: The three keys to change at work and life.* New York: HarperCollins.

Miller, W., & Rollnick, S. (2002). *Motivational interviewing: preparing people for change.* New York: Guilford Press.

Norcross, J., & Loeberg, K. (2013). *Changeology: 5 steps to realizing your goals and resolutions.* New York: Simon and Schuster.

Prochaska, J. O., & DiClemente, C. C. (1983). Stages and process of self-change of smoking: Toward an integrative model of change. *Journal of Consulting and Clinical Psychology, 51*(3), 390–395.

Willis, J., & Frye Campbell, L. (1992). *Exercise psychology.* Champaign, IL: Human Kinetics.

# CHAPTER 8

# Client Assessment

*"It takes a lot of courage to show your dreams to someone else."*

—ERMA BOMBECK

**OBJECTIVES**

**After reading this chapter, you will be able to:**

- Identify the value of assessments to the coaching partnership
- Identify assessments to use with clients
- Review a sample well-being assessment
- Identify medical or mental health red flags
- Prepare for and support a first coaching session

## The Value of Assessments

Client assessments are valuable tools in the coach's toolbox and offer a variety of benefits to the coaching partnership.

In the corporate environment, an executive or business coach might measure behaviors and ways of being using assessments of emotional intelligence (EI) or personality type. Coaches of various niches may use a variety of assessments focused on life balance or wellness. A common example is the "wheel of life," which is focused on self-care and balance. Assessments of character strengths or talents provide an excellent springboard for new directions in coaching sessions. Many coaches

and clinical groups value the positivity ratio. The higher the ratio, the more resources available for change, and increasing the ratio is a valuable goal.

Assessments stimulate reflection and self-awareness. Assessments can be helpful at the beginning of a coaching relationship because they not only inform coaches, they also help clients gain self-awareness, insights, and a sense of their priorities for a coaching program. Assessments are also efficient because precious coaching time isn't used to gather a lot of data; that can feel like an interrogation.

Other benefits of having clients complete an assessment include:

1. Trust and rapport: When building trust with a new client, an online or paper assessment provides him or her with a safe space in which to first tell his or her "story."
2. Honoring personality preferences: Clients with a preference for introversion will tend to be more comfortable communicating personal information in writing, at least initially, than those with a more extroverted preference.
3. The written word: There is power in providing clients with an opportunity to see

a qualitative and quantitative summary of their state of well-being. For the same reasons that writing down goals is important, seeing the information collectively can be both affirming and a powerful motivator for action.

4. Developing discrepancy: An assessment can help a client more clearly see the difference between where they are and where they are not in terms of behaviors and outcomes.

The process of deliberately answering questions about subjects such as one's priorities, needs, values, readiness, and challenges promotes self-discovery and expands awareness. By stimulating such mindful noticing, assessments begin the coaching process even before the first coaching session. People become more aware of who they are, where they are starting, what well-being encompasses, and where they want to go. The International Coach Federation (2014) identifies "creating awareness" as a core coaching competency precisely because awareness precedes action in the service of goals.

Progress depends on clients expanding their awareness of what is possible. This cannot be done *for* them without provoking resistance. They must do it for themselves, and assessments are an excellent way to get the conversation started. Through listening, inquiry, and reflections, coaches can then expand client awareness even further in the process of assisting clients in climbing Mount Lasting Change. At its best, ever-expanding awareness generates an upward spiral of continuous learning, growth, and development.

When coaches are integrated into healthcare, corporate wellness, or health promotion programs, tracking health behavioral and biometric data through assessments is vital for program outcomes measurement. Health risk assessments (HRAs), such as the one provided at vectorwellness.com, are now widely validated and used as tools by health plans and employers to measure health and lifestyle status as well as change readiness. These also may identify "red flags" with respect to mental health status or medical care gaps.

Assessments are invaluable to coaches in the health and wellness fields because they can provide:

- An overall picture of the client's present state of being including physical health, lifestyle habits, strengths, life satisfaction, and readiness to make changes
- A snapshot to better understand and appreciate the client's life context; the coaching questions and approach for a client who has significant health issues such as obesity, hypertension, back injury, or cancer is different than the approach for a highly motivated, fit client
- Awareness of situations, such as a major loss or recent diagnosis
- Early indication of the client's strengths and healthy habits as well as health risks and areas of challenge
- Identification of red flags related to physical health issues (e.g., medical care gaps, injury, or contraindications to exercise) or mental health issues (depression or other mental health concerns) for which a referral may be important or even critical

## A Caution in the Use of Assessments

Although assessments are valuable when used appropriately with the best of coaching skills, there are still a few potential dangers which we explore below.

### Less Room for Collaboration and More Room for the Expert Hat

If a coach is not well-trained in using an appreciative approach to reviewing and debriefing results, assessments tend to shine the light on what is "wrong" in client behaviors and outcomes. It can be tempting to fall into old habits of looking for what needs to be fixed and donning the "expert hat" to do so right away. Noticing biometric numbers that need to go up or down, for example, could shift a health coach into "fix it" mode, listing all of the dangers and "shoulds" for a client. Although being aware of health concerns and other concerns is vitally important, a masterful coach uses an assessment as a conduit for deeper conversations rather than as a mandate for prescribing change.

### Evaluation Rather than Empathy

When an assessment reveals a client's health or life choices are of concern, it can be tempting to experience pity or sympathy for the client. Frustration can emerge as the coach wonders how the client could have chosen a particular behavior, such as smoking, overeating, or overworking. Instead of evaluation, assessments can provide an opportunity to show acceptance and express empathy. The review of and conversation surrounding an assessment can establish the foundation of trust between coach and client that lays the groundwork for the growth-promoting relationship.

### Assessments Are Completed by Humans

Lastly, assessments are completed by people who get distracted, do them at the last minute, and/or mark responses to please or impress their coaches. Hence, assessments aren't always accurate and don't tell the whole story. The coaching session is the place for the assessment to come to life through reflection, inquiry, and listening.

The bottom line is that concern for compassion should always come before concern for compliance in any coaching relationship and not just because it feels better; compassion leads to more behavioral change (Jack, Boyatzis, Khawaja, Passarelli, & Leckie, 2013). Although compliance-based conversations activate the sympathetic nervous system (which is activated when a person senses danger), coaching-based conversations activate the parasympathetic nervous system which enables problem solving, envisioning, and taking a view of a broader perspective.

### Assessments and Autonomy

Most importantly, when used with a coaching approach, assessments are a tool to uncover the motivational drivers for the clients, indicating what is most important to them and the priorities they have for their lives. Assessments can be an excellent strategy for ensuring that the client feels in control of the process, competent to make progress, and in a relationship with a compassionate coach partner on the journey.

## Assessments for Coaching

There are many assessments that coaches use, initially or during the coaching relationship to support the client in creating greater self-awareness as well as a vision and goals. The following list includes assessments, or assessment methodologies, that coaches in a variety of domains find helpful in their work with clients.

1. *Six Dimensions of Wellness*: Dr. Bill Hettler (1976), co-founder of the U.S. National Wellness Institute, developed the six dimensions of wellness model (Fig. 8.1), defining wellness as an active process through which people become aware of and make choices toward a more successful existence: contribution, connection, values, self-care, self-determination, and contribution.

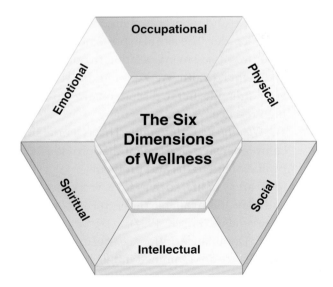

**Figure 8.1.** The Six Dimensions of Wellness (Hettler, 1976).

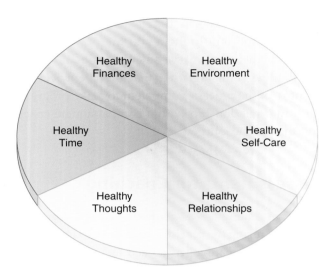

**Figure 8.2.** The Wheel of Life.

2. *The Wheel of Life*: Using the Wheel of Life (Fig. 8.2), a concept made popular in *Coactive Coaching* (Kimsey-House, Kimsey-House, Sandahl, & Whitworth, 2011), clients rate their levels of satisfaction in each area using a scale of 0–10 with 10 being total satisfaction. The center of the wheel represents 0 and the outer edge is 10.

3. *Values-in-Action (VIA) Signature Strengths Questionnaire*: The VIA Signature Strengths Questionnaire is a free 240-question assessment (Peterson & Seligman, 2004) that measures and reports 24 character strengths in rank order. The site also hosts numerous other free assessments relating to optimism and mental health. We explored the 24 character strengths in the discussion on "Coaching Presence."

4. *The Quality of Life Inventory*: This is a brief but comprehensive assessment that provides a profile of strengths and problems in 16 areas of life, such as love, work, health, and play. It is available through Pearson Assessments (Frisch, 1994).

5. *DISC*: Dominance, influence, steadiness, and compliance are examined in this four-quadrant behavioral model that examines the behavior of individuals in their environment or within a specific situation. DISC looks at behavioral styles and preferences (Clarke, 1976).

6. *Myers Briggs Type Indicator*: One of the most widely used and highly respected measures of personality preferences; it identifies individual preferences in terms of four pairs of preferences: extroversion–introversion, sensing–intuition, thinking–feeling, and judging–perceiving (Myers & Briggs, 1975). In her book, *8 Colors of Fitness,* author Suzanne Brue (2008) asserts by understanding type preferences, clients can understand their fitness personality. With this understanding, they can choose the specific forms, interactions, and environments that are most appropriate for them.

7. *Positivity Ratio*: Based on the work of Dr. Barbara Fredrickson (2009), the score provides a snapshot of how one's emotions of the past day combine to create your positivity ratio, the ratio of positive emotions to negative emotions.

8. *Self-Compassion Scale*: From Kristin Neff's (2011) definition of compassion (self-kindness, a sense of common humanity, and mindfulness), this assessment provides insight into one's level of self-compassion.

9. *Mindful Attention Awareness Scale (MAAS)*: The MAAS, validated by Brown and Ryan (2003), examines openness and receptive awareness to what is taking place in the moment.

10. *Five Facet Mindfulness Scale*: Another exploration of mindfulness based on observing, describing, acting with awareness, nonjudging of inner experience, and non-reactivity to inner experience (Baer, Smith, Hopkins, Krietemeyer, & Toney, 2006)

11. *Quickie Well-Being Assessment*: A short-form questionnaire development by Wellcoaches focused on foundational areas of well-being (Moore, 2011) (Fig. 8.3)

12. *Decisional Balance*: As introduced in a previous chapter, motivational interviewing is a methodology that supports the eliciting of autonomous motivation, encouraging

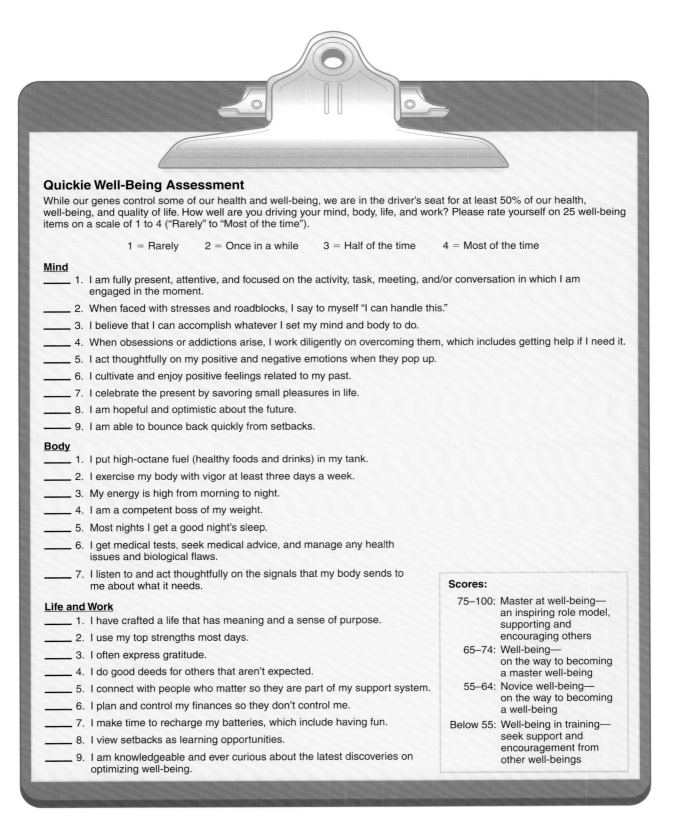

## Quickie Well-Being Assessment

While our genes control some of our health and well-being, we are in the driver's seat for at least 50% of our health, well-being, and quality of life. How well are you driving your mind, body, life, and work? Please rate yourself on 25 well-being items on a scale of 1 to 4 ("Rarely" to "Most of the time").

1 = Rarely    2 = Once in a while    3 = Half of the time    4 = Most of the time

### Mind

_____ 1. I am fully present, attentive, and focused on the activity, task, meeting, and/or conversation in which I am engaged in the moment.

_____ 2. When faced with stresses and roadblocks, I say to myself "I can handle this."

_____ 3. I believe that I can accomplish whatever I set my mind and body to do.

_____ 4. When obsessions or addictions arise, I work diligently on overcoming them, which includes getting help if I need it.

_____ 5. I act thoughtfully on my positive and negative emotions when they pop up.

_____ 6. I cultivate and enjoy positive feelings related to my past.

_____ 7. I celebrate the present by savoring small pleasures in life.

_____ 8. I am hopeful and optimistic about the future.

_____ 9. I am able to bounce back quickly from setbacks.

### Body

_____ 1. I put high-octane fuel (healthy foods and drinks) in my tank.

_____ 2. I exercise my body with vigor at least three days a week.

_____ 3. My energy is high from morning to night.

_____ 4. I am a competent boss of my weight.

_____ 5. Most nights I get a good night's sleep.

_____ 6. I get medical tests, seek medical advice, and manage any health issues and biological flaws.

_____ 7. I listen to and act thoughtfully on the signals that my body sends to me about what it needs.

### Life and Work

_____ 1. I have crafted a life that has meaning and a sense of purpose.

_____ 2. I use my top strengths most days.

_____ 3. I often express gratitude.

_____ 4. I do good deeds for others that aren't expected.

_____ 5. I connect with people who matter so they are part of my support system.

_____ 6. I plan and control my finances so they don't control me.

_____ 7. I make time to recharge my batteries, which include having fun.

_____ 8. I view setbacks as learning opportunities.

_____ 9. I am knowledgeable and ever curious about the latest discoveries on optimizing well-being.

**Scores:**

75–100: Master at well-being—an inspiring role model, supporting and encouraging others

65–74: Well-being—on the way to becoming a master well-being

55–64: Novice well-being—on the way to becoming a well-being

Below 55: Well-being in training—seek support and encouragement from other well-beings

**Figure 8.3.** The Quickie Well-Being Assessment.

a client to find his or her own reasons to change. It involves pro-change talk and avoids triggering of change-resistance talk, which can cause the client to resist being told what to do. Through the use of motivational interviewing techniques, such the Decisional Balance Tool, coaches and clients review reasons for and against change as a tool for assessing readiness to change (Botelho, 2008). Coaches also ask clients to assess readiness, willingness, and ability to change using rulers on a scale of 0–10.

13. *Transtheoretical Model of Change*: The five stages of change model provide coaches with an understanding of how and when new health-promoting behaviors can be adopted and sustained and why clients may struggle, fail, or quit (Prochaska, Norcross, & DiClemente, 1994). Assessing the client's stage of change for a particular behavior is critical for identifying appropriate change strategies.

## A Well-Being Assessment

Wellcoaches developed a comprehensive well-being assessment built on concepts developed by Dee Edington, PhD (2008), a leading health promotion researcher while at the University of Michigan. Edington is also a developer of an industry standard health risk appraisal. The assessment is online and serves to enhance the client's self-awareness and provide foundational information for the coach. As a holistic assessment, it looks at the many different components of well-being, including:

1. *Energy*: levels of energy throughout a typical day, including energy boosters and energy drains

2. *Life satisfaction*: sense of purpose, joy, gratitude, work satisfaction, and personal relationship satisfaction

3. *Mental and emotional fitness*: coping skills, resilience, sleep patterns, stress levels, emotional status, social activity/support, and personal loss

4. *Weight management*: body mass index, height, weight, and waist measurement

5. *Physical activity/exercise*: frequency and types of physical activity

6. *Nutrition*: intake frequency of healthy snacks, whole grains, fruits and vegetables, water, soft drinks, alcoholic beverages, and trans fats

7. *Health*: blood pressure, cholesterol, heart rate, relationship with a physician, gender-related health issues, frequency of illness, medications, tobacco use, and personal/family health history

Clients find it especially valuable to look at wellness from this broader perspective, acknowledging that energy, life satisfaction, and mental/emotional fitness are key contributors to health in addition to the "traditional" factors such as weight and nutrition.

## Uncovering Motivation

This well-being assessment can provide initial information about a client's:

1. *Priorities*: An assessment can be designed to calculate or allow clients to indicate their areas of highest priority. For example, on a scale of 0–10 (10 being the highest), the client may indicate that focusing the coaching program on improving life satisfaction is a 10 (highest priority), whereas improving nutritional habits is a 5 (of average priority).

2. *Confidence*: Similarly, the assessment may include a method for clients to indicate the strength of their belief in their ability to make a behavioral change. This information enables the coach to more appropriately design opportunities for the development of *self-efficacy* by working with the appropriate personal, environmental, and behavioral factors.

3. *Readiness for change*: It is beneficial for an assessment to create an awareness of the client's *stage of change* within the various areas. When it comes to moving a client forward,

each of the five stages of change (*precontemplation, contemplation, preparation, action, and maintenance*) requires a different approach for exploration. Knowing where a client stands in terms of their readiness is critical for setting goals that are appropriate to the client's stage of change and for building self-efficacy.

## Explore Assessment Results

A protocol for the appreciative review and exploration of client assessments is described below. Although this protocol was developed for the review of wellness, well-being, health, and HRAs, the principles are relevant to other assessments too.

1. *Read with an open mind.* Prior to the first coaching session, take time to carefully review the client's completed assessment. In reviewing, the goal is not to evaluate but to consider the responses with curiosity, keeping in mind that an assessment provides only a partial story. Open-minded curiosity will enable the coach to ask better questions during the assessment review, use intuition and sense what is unsaid, challenge the coach's assumptions about the client, develop a strengths-based framework through which to appreciate the client, and be more open to new information and energy shifts during the first coaching session.

2. *Seek out success.* It is tempting to begin an assessment review with a search for all of the "problems" or areas to "fix." Drawing on the lessons from the disciplines of appreciative inquiry and positive psychology, we know that "what we focus on grows" and that "our first questions are fateful." Therefore, if the coach begins the initial review of the client's information with a focus on what's "wrong," an assessment is more likely to support that tendency within coaching relationships. Starting with the assumption that all clients can tap into capacities and leverage strengths for positive change will enable the coach to better support clients in the building of self-efficacy.

3. *Notice the client's arousal.* The next task in reviewing a client's assessment is to look for the areas in which the client is feeling an emotional charge, either positive or negative. Look for places in which the client indicates there is a concentrated energy, such as in his or her priorities for change and the importance he or she assigns to each of the well-being areas. The role of the coach is to look for the client's autonomous motivation—the areas in which the client is expressing an interest in growth and change—not the areas in which the coach believes the client should be interested.

4. *Consider the stages of change.* If the assessment includes indicators of the client's stage(s) of change, consider how this might impact the coaching program and the client's needs. Remember to prioritize the cognitive and emotional goals in the early stages of change and the planning and action goals in the later stages of change.

5. *Question gaps.* Due to design or user errors or incomplete answers, assessments will sometimes leave the coach with questions about inconsistencies in responses. For example, a client may name improving nutrition as the "highest priority" while indicating a low score in terms of readiness to change. In these cases, the coach will want to take note and be prepared to inquire about the discrepancy in information during the coaching session.

6. *Note concerns.* Where appropriate, an assessment review should include an examination of any mental health or medical concerns indicated by the client. Be aware of any red flags such as health risks, injuries, or other health concerns that might require a physician's release before engaging in regular exercise. If a client wants exercise to be a part of the coaching program, a physician release form can be provided to the client to give to his or her physician. This is a document the coach can create, asking the client's doctor for any recommendations or restrictions in working with a coach.

Guidelines pertaining to the need for medical clearance and exercise participation are available from organizations such as the American College of Sports Medicine (ACSM, 2013) in their *ACSM's Guidelines for Exercise Testing and Prescription*. Guidelines for nutrition can be found through the Academy of Nutrition and Dietetics, Centers for Disease Control and Prevention (CDC) Healthy Living site, and www.nutritionfacts.org. Coaches without recognized education and experience in these areas should always refer to an expert or expert sources.

## COACHING CASE

**Wendy Well:** "I have diabetes and I was considering not taking my medicine because I think it makes me feel worse. If our coaching helps me make better food choices, I think I'll probably stop taking the medicine."

**Coach Carl:** "It can be frustrating when you're taking medications that make you feel worse than better in some ways. And you have hope that changing your diet will help you feel better so that one day you may not need medication. However, I am not a physician or a dietitian, so those decisions are beyond the scope of our work together, and I cannot advise you on that topic. As you are working with a medical doctor for this, I recommend that you continue to seek the recommendations of your doctor and that you have your physician complete a release for us to work together safely."

Although coaches do not diagnose mental health risks, they need to know what to look for in order to make appropriate recommendations or referrals to a psychologist, therapist, or physician for consultation. The following indicators are examples and not all inclusive:

- *Depression*: Clients who are not eating or sleeping in normal patterns, such as not sleeping or sleeping all of the time, appetite loss, or binge eating, may be showing signs of clinical depression and may need to be referred to their physicians.
- *Eating disorders*: Clients who have lost a great deal of weight without surgery and/or medication and continue to do so when advised it will be harmful to their health (anorexia), exercise beyond their normal physical capacity, or continue to gain and/or lose 20–30 pounds without stabilizing, may be showing signs of an eating disorder and may need to be referred to their physicians.
- *Substance abuse*: Clients who display unusual behaviors, such as acting out or violent outbursts, that are uncharacteristic of their usual behaviors may be showing signs of substance abuse, including steroid use, and may need to be referred to their physicians.
- *Anxiety disorders*: Clients who suffer from panic attacks, claustrophobic behavior, or shortness of breath may be showing signs of anxiety disorder and may need to be referred to their physicians.

If a client shares a serious or life-threatening mental or physical health issue during an assessment or coaching session, advise him or her that the situation is outside of the scope of coaching and encourage and assist him or her to seek professional help as soon as possible.

## Honor Intuition and the Client

If a coach has a sense that a client should seek further medical attention or needs resources outside the coach's expertise, a coach must respectfully express that concern. If the client then chooses not to engage with additional resources, it is recommended that the coaching relationship be terminated until the client has received the appropriate assistance. Therefore, it is valuable to build relationships with highly respected health experts that could serve as sources for referrals. This may also lead to cross-referrals and business building. If a coach does not have connections to appropriate referrals, clients can also be encouraged to see their primary care physicians for referrals.

If a coach seeks advice about a client from another health professional, it is critical that the tenets of the Health Insurance Portability and Accountability Act (HIPAA) are followed, taking full precautions not to share the client's name or any revealing personal information (US Department of Health and Human Services).

## Coaching with a Well-Being Assessment

The first coaching sessions with a client are an opportunity for establishing trust and rapport, confirming a coach's sense of the client's circumstances based on any assessments that may have been completed ahead of time and determining the readiness/energy level of the client for change. It should never be assumed that assessments completed ahead of time reveal the whole story or reflect how the client will be feeling when the coaching session takes place. Also, mistakes or misinterpretation of questions can sometimes occur when filling out forms.

It is wise to confirm in a coaching session important items that might be significant in working toward a client's vision or checking in on items that don't seem to add up based on other comments. That's why it's so important for coaches to practice mindfulness and to be in the moment with clients rather than fixated on the results of an assessment. Assessments are helpful as guides; they become unhelpful when they introduce an agenda that triggers a client to become resistant.

## Establish Trust and Rapport

It is crucial to establish trust and rapport with clients at the outset of every coaching session; that is especially true at the outset of the first coaching session. Coach and client may be unknown to each other apart from information exchanged ahead of time, so it is essential for coaches to put clients at ease and to bring them into their confidence through:

- Holding clients in positive regard
- Expressing empathy
- Slowing down
- Listening with full attention

- Allowing clients to formulate and find their own answers
- Honestly sharing observations
- Under-promising and over-delivering
- Being humble in sharing information and advice
- Honoring confidentiality

## Uncover Motivation

The coach begins by thanking the client for completing the assessment(s), and get a sense of their experience and learning from assessments. Ask the client to share any feelings, issues, or questions they may have in the wake of the assessment(s). Pay attention to the emotional charge as well to the underlying needs so that you can offer an empathetic reflection in reply. It is important that the client feels heard and respected on an emotional level before moving on.

- "What's most important for you right now?"
- "What are you most excited to talk about?"
- "What are you yearning for in your life?"
- "What areas of life make you feel most alive?"

These are the operative inquiries. Regardless of how they may have rated and prioritized things at the time of the assessment(s), coaches work with clients in the moment. Things may have shifted between then and now for any number of reasons (including the taking of the assessment[s] themselves). It's the job of the coach to remain open to the presenting energy and issues of the client rather than showing up with an agenda for the coaching session (however grounded that may be in the assessments). The aim is to flow and co-construct things with the client rather than to wear the expert hat of teacher or advisor.

## Use Appreciative Inquiry to Discover Client Successes, Strengths, Frameworks, and Hopes

The best way to discuss an assessment is to use the information gleaned from it to make powerful, client-specific, strength-based inquiries in a way that will assist clients in knowing themselves and moving forward in the direction of their desired futures. By asking clients open-ended questions about their successes, strengths, frameworks, and hopes, the coach will not only learn more about their priorities and the issues they want to focus on at this time, but it will also elevate the client's readiness and energy for change. Clients are used to taking assessments that have the intention of revealing flaws that need to be fixed; it is refreshing when assessments are used to reveal strengths that need to be reinforced. Conversations about assessments are a time for learning rather than telling what clients should know or do.

Other inquiries are:

- "What questions do you have after completing the assessment?"
- "What insights do you have by completing the assessment?"
- "I'm curious about the way you responded to ... Tell me more."
- "About what do you feel most proud?"
- "What surprised you?"
- "What concerns you? "

Masterful coaching is about paying attention to and building on the energy clients show up with for coaching. When their energy is low (whether physically, mentally, emotionally, or spiritually), appreciative empathy can bring new energy. When their energy is high, appreciative inquiry can assist them with getting or staying inspired. Either way, discovering client successes, strengths, frameworks, and hopes that are grounded in reality as revealed by the assessment(s) and by what they have to say now, in the moment, will enable clients to develop a vision and to design appropriate actions.

## Discover Preferred Client Learning Modes and Styles

People learn best in different ways. More than 80 learning style models have been developed and another book would be needed to do them justice. The Myers Briggs and DISC assessments, to mention only two of the more popular ones, reveal learning styles and are among the models to consider. Although there is considerable criticism of the validity of learning style models and assessments by psychologists and psychometricians, there is no dispute that individual preferences in learning styles play a role in change and learning. Take weight loss, for example. Some prefer to learn from books, some want a close personal mentor such as a personal trainer, some enjoy online self-help programs or online social networks, some value a local live group discussion or class format, some seek out competitions, whereas others do best when they go away for an intensive learning week with experts.

One of the International Coach Federation's (2014) core coaching competencies relates to learning style: "[The coach] demonstrates respect for client's perceptions, learning style, and personal being." Apart from such respect, it's important for clients to connect with coaches in ways that promote their learning and growth. Noticing the language and approaches they use, the coach can then better come alongside clients in the process of enabling them to more rapidly and successfully acquire new knowledge and skills.

## Discuss Components of the Assessment

Next, the coach will inform the client that they have reviewed their assessments ahead of time, getting a sense of where they are at right now and on what they want to work. Explain, however, that assessments never tell the whole story and that it would be helpful if they would be willing to share what surfaced for them during the assessment and where they want to go with what emerged. Ask specific questions to clarify missing information and to bolster the self-confidence of the client. Seek out successes to notice the client's emotional charge, identify the client's readiness to change, and note concerns that may relate to physical or mental health risks.

When clients talk about "failures" or things that have not worked for them in the past, a coach can support them in reframing those experiences as learning opportunities and life lessons. Clients grow through "trial and correction," not "trial and error." By taking this non-judgmental, growth-oriented framework, coaches create a safe place in which clients can open up and say anything. Whenever possible, the coach can champion a client's capacity to change and assisting him or her in finding compelling reasons to try again.

Curiosity on the part of a coach empowers clients to find their own answers, to be more resourceful, and to discover new possibilities for moving forward. Curiosity is not interrogation; it is rather an open, inviting, judgment-free, leisurely, and even playful exploration of opportunities for learning and growth. As the coach demonstrates curiosity with the clients, the clients will be more curious about their own capacities and more willing to try new things.

To use curiosity well, a coach uses deep, open-ended inquiries that require thought to answer and connect clients to their heartfelt dreams and desires. Such questions often reveal information that would not otherwise come to the surface. It is important to:

- Notice the energy shifts in client responses.
- Be curious when there is a change in affect, whether that's increased energy for change or resistance to it.
- Avoid responding to clients with analytical questions. For example, if a client says, "I want to lose weight" or "I need to get in shape" say "Tell me about what makes that important to you" or "Tell me about what that would make possible for you." Such curiosity is likely to elicit more information than "Why do you want to do that?" because analytical "why" questions can sound challenging or judgmental.

Related to an assessment such as the Wellcoaches well-being assessment, questions such as the following are useful in generating deeper insights:

- **Personal**
  - You mentioned that you have children/grandchildren. Tell me about them.
  - What brought you to a coach?
  - What would be different in your life if you felt healthier and fit?
- **Physical activity**
  - What fitness activities did you like in the past?
  - What fitness activities can you see yourself doing?

- I noticed from your assessment that you haven't exercised recently. Tell me about that.
- **Nutrition**
  - What healthy eating habits do you have now?
  - What changes would you like to make in your eating?
  - How do you feel about your eating right now?
  - What eating habits would you like to improve?
- **Weight management**
  - When have you been the most successful at managing your weight? Describe your experience and the circumstances.
  - You said you weigh "X" now, and you'd like to weigh "Y." What would that change make possible?
  - Tell me about your best past experiences with weight management.
  - What has worked in the past?
  - What have you learned from your past efforts in managing weight that would be helpful in the future?
- **Stress**
  - When is your stress at its lowest?
  - What works best for you when it comes to managing stress?
  - What do you do when you're under stress?
  - What have you tried in the past to reduce stress that would be helpful in the future?
- **Energy**
  - How would you describe your daily energy level?
  - What fills your cup and gives you energy?
  - What empties your cup and drains your energy?
- **Health**
  - When was the last time you had a physical exam with a physician?
  - How are you feeling today?
  - Tell me about your relationship with your physician.
  - I see from your questionnaire that you have [name of condition]. What is the treatment plan you have been following?
  - What is your greatest hope related to your health?

- **Life satisfaction**
  - What are you most satisfied about in your life?
  - For what are you most grateful?
  - What brings you the most pleasure?
- **Other possible inquiries include the following:**
  - What are you doing presently in this area of health, fitness, and wellness?
  - Describe your best experience with this area.
  - What have you done in the past that worked?
  - How would you rate your mastery of this area on a scale of 0–10?
  - By what values are you striving to live by?
  - How are your environment, work, and relationships impacting you?
  - Tell me more about . . .

## References

American College of Sports Medicine. (2013). *ACSM's guidelines for exercise testing and prescription* (9th ed.). Lippincott Williams & Wilkins.

Baer, R. A., Smith, G. T., Hopkins, J., Krietemeyer, J., & Toney, L. (2006). Using self-report assessment methods to explore facets of mindfulness. *Assessment, 13,* 27–45.

Botelho, R. (2008). *Motivate healthy habits: Stepping stones to lasting change.* Rochester, NY: MHH Publications.

Brown, K., & Ryan, R. (2003). The benefits of being present: Mindfulness and its role in psychological well-being. *Journal of Personality and Social Psychology, 84*(4), 822–848.

Brue, S. (2008). *The 8 colors of fitness: Discover your color-coded fitness personality and create an exercise program you'll never quit!* Burlington, VT: Oakledge Press.

Clarke, W. (1976). DISC. Retrieved April 27, 2015 from https://www.discprofile.com/what-is-disc/history-of-disc/ Published by Inscape Publishing.

Edintgon, D. (2008). *Health risk assessment.* Retrieved October 29, 2008 from http://www.hmrc.umich.edu/services/HRA%20092007.pdf

Fredrickson, B. (2009). *Positivity: Groundbreaking research reveals how to embrace the hidden strength of positive emotions, overcome negativity, and thrive.* New York: Crown.

Frisch, M. B. (1994). *Quality of life inventory manual and treatment guide.* Minneapolis, MN: NCS Pearson and Pearson Assessments.

Hettler, B. (1976). *Six dimensions of wellness.* Retrieved April 27, 2015 from http://www.nationalwellness.org/?page=Six_Dimensions

International Coach Federation. *Core competencies.* Retrieved March 25, 2014 from http://coachfederation.org/credential/landing.cfm?ItemNumber=2206&navItemNumber=576

Jack, A., Boyatzis, R., Khawaja, M., Passarelli, A., & Leckie, R. (2013). Visioning in the brain: An fMRI study of inspirational coaching and mentoring. *Social Neuroscience, 8,* 369–384.

Kimsey-House, H., Kimsey-House, K., Sandahl, P., & Whitworth, L. (2011). *Co-active coaching.* Boston, MA: Nicholas Brealey America.

Moore, M. (2011). *Quickie well-being assessment.* Wellesley, MA: Wellcoaches.

Myers, I., & Briggs, K. (1975). *Myers Briggs type inventory.* Mountain View, CA: CPP.

Neff, K. (2011). *Self-compassion: The proven power of being kind to yourself.* New York: William Morrow.

Peterson, C., & Seligman, M. E. P. (2004). *Character strengths and virtues: A handbook and classification.* Washington, DC: American Psychological Association.

Prochaska, J. O., Norcross, J. C., & DiClemente, C. C. (1994). *Changing for good.* New York: HarperCollins.

# CHAPTER 9

# Design Thinking

*"Goals are dreams with deadlines."*

—DIANA SCHARF HUNT

## OBJECTIVES

**After reading this chapter, you will be able to:**

- Describe design thinking and its connection to coaching
- Describe the process of designing a coaching agreement with the client
- Describe the process of designing a vision within a coaching session
- Describe the process of designing three-month and weekly goals within a coaching session

## Introduction to Planning

There are few human endeavors that succeed without investing the time and effort to develop realistic and inspiring plans. In the workplace, planning is the basis for forward progress, change, and transformation. Accordingly, planning and goal setting are among the International Coach Federation's (2014) core coaching competencies. Realistic and inspiring plans also provide the framework for clients to improve their health and wellness.

Wellcoaches has designed and refined a visioning, planning, and goal setting process for coaches to use with clients: well-suited but not limited to the journey toward mastery of health and well-being. Not only does it assist clients in establishing new life habits and making behavioral changes that last, clients also learn life skills that enable change and build the capacity for future change. Coaches assist clients in developing well-conceived plans through the creation of a compelling vision—one that strongly beckons—three-month goals designed to lead to that vision, and weekly behavioral goals that generate steady and incremental progress.

## The Nature of Design Thinking

Design thinking, a concept born of the world of architects and artists, provides some important principles for co-creating plans with coaching clients. Like architects, coaches support clients in creating a clear vision of what they want to build and help make plans to create strong foundations and frameworks on which to build. In the design process, the coach as "architect" takes a solution-focused approach, incorporating both analysis and imagination. According to Nelson and Stolterman (2012), "Design is the action of bringing something new and desired into existence—a proactive stance that resolves or dissolves problematic situations by design."

This collaborative state requires open-ended inquiry, mindful listening, and empathy above all. The coach as "designer" doesn't come to the design stage with a predetermined idea of what the client's vision and goals should be. Instead, coaches honor the principles of design that rely on the following strategies (Brown, 2008):

*Empathy.* Seeing the world through the eyes of the client by encouraging the client to tell his or her own story and listening for the perspectives the client has to share. The coach listens for the spoken and unspoken, checking out intuitions and tapping into the creativity of client.

*Optimism.* The coach assumes that no matter how challenging the constraints of the client's situation, there is always a solution, and the client is capable of success. Much like the anticipatory principle of appreciative inquiry, a coach who uses design thinking holds a positive image of the future on behalf of the client.

*Collaboration.* The design thinking approach acknowledges the value of the collaborative nature of inspiration and design. Similar to the constructionist principle of appreciative inquiry and lessons learned from social cognitive theory, there is recognition of the power of two or more brains working toward a grand design which, in the case of coaching, is the grand design for one's life!

*Experimentalism.* "Significant innovations don't come from incremental tweaks. Design thinkers pose questions and explore constraints in creative ways that proceed in entirely new directions," states Brown (2008). In the process of creating a great vision and subsequent goals, this means that both coach and client must let go of the idea that the first idea is the best idea. This opens up the opportunity for prototype testing, evaluation, and redesign along the way.

## Designing the Coaching Program

The startup of a coaching program sets the tone for the entire coaching relationship both by establishing trust and rapport and by creating an inspiring and engaging vision and goals on which a client will work for weeks and months to come. The design of the relationship—including the principles of empathy, positivity, creative collaboration, and a learning and growth mindset through experimentation—is ideally conveyed to the client at the outset.

## Designing the Coaching Agreement

The first session is an opportunity to ask a few "get to know you" questions related to the client's occupation, family, hobbies, physical activities, or daily routine and to find areas of commonality between coach and client. The coach can briefly share his or her own biography but should avoid talking too long or too much about him or herself so as not to take the focus off of the client and the client's agenda for coaching.

It is also an opportunity to convey the coach's heartfelt passion about the work as well as to describe relevant education and experience. Clients can tell when the coach is reciting lines, and it does not sound genuine. Before beginning the coaching session, ask "What more do you want to know about me before we begin?"

Of course, the underlying reason for these "warm up" conversations is to establish a sense of connection between coach and client. Humans have a need to belong, which includes a perception that the other feels a genuine concern and has a long-term interest in being connected (Baumeister & Leary, 1995). For client's to become self-determining beings, they need to feel connected to others and experience a sense of belonging "with" another (Deci & Ryan, 2002). The coaching relationship is above all a collaborative partnership with deep respect for the talents, strengths, and skills that each person brings to it.

## Describe the Role of the Coach

The first session is a critical time to explain or remind the client of the difference between education and coaching. Whereas educators have information, expertise, and wisdom that they want to share with their students, coaches enable clients to discover a lot of that for themselves. On occasion and when appropriate, coaches may provide expert advice or knowledge during a coaching session (Wolever et al., 2013). Most of the time, however, coaches will listen, ask questions, and reflect what they are hearing in ways that promote client learning, growth, and movement. That is the coach approach—it's a personalized learning system which enables clients to find their own answers and achieve exceptional results even in the face of challenges. The coach can share his or her confidence that this approach often assists clients in reaching higher than they would otherwise. It is even better when this confidence is based on a coach's track record of client success.

## There Is No One "Right" Way

It is crucial that clients realize they are not getting a cookie-cutter approach. With regard to supporting a client's autonomy and competence, the kind of connection that grows out of coaching relationship is the kind that is organically shaped based on the present needs of the client. A masterful coach does not apply a "one-size-fits-all" template to the client moving through the change process. This is why masterful coaches rely on a variety of theories and processes, such as self-determination (Deci & Ryan, 1985); positive psychology (Peterson, 2006); appreciative inquiry (Cooperrider & Whitney, 2005); nonviolent communication (Rosenberg, 2005); motivational interviewing (Miller & Rollnick, 2012); emotional intelligence (Goleman, 1996); design thinking (Brown, 2008); and flow theory (Csikszentmihalyi, 1990). No single model can provide all of the tools needed to support the complexity of the dynamics of change in human beings impacted by a multitude of factors within their psyches and in their environments. Coaches spend a lifetime adding to their toolboxes in order to continually improve their client outcomes.

## Highlight the Promise to Build and Maintain Trust

One of the most crucial ways to build trust is through responsible and respectful record keeping. Being clear about policies of confidentiality and record keeping assures that coaches respect the client's right to privacy and are fundamentally prudent in the protection of those rights (within the limits of institutional regulations and/or laws such as the Health Insurance Portability and Accountability Act) (U.S. Department of Health and Human Services, 2014). This extends to those records created, stored, accessed, transferred, and disposed of by coaches during the course of working with clients. Clients base their trust in a coach on the assessment of the coach's benevolence, honesty, openness, reliability, and competence (Tschannen-Moran, 2004). The coach's commitment to maintaining confidentiality is key to maintaining this trust.

## Agree on Coaching Principles

It is important for coaches and clients to agree and commit to some key principles for coaching programs before or during the first coaching session (Whitworth, Kimsey-House, Kimsey-House, & Sandhal, 2007).

For example, the coach and client may consider agreeing on the following principles at the onset of the coaching relationship:

### Coach

- I will help my client identify and fully engage his or her strengths on the path to a better future.
- I will ask provocative questions and encourage my client to arrive at his or her own answers whenever possible and co-create answers otherwise.
- I will encourage realistic expectations and goals.
- I will be direct and firm with constructive reflections when needed.
- I will support my client in brainstorming creative possibilities for moving forward and navigating roadblocks.
- When appropriate, with permission, and within my scope of practice, I will offer advice,

instruction, and resources for improving health, well-being, and performance.

- I will be punctual and responsive.
- I will recognize early whether the chemistry with a client is good or not optimal. If not optimal, I will refer the client to another coach.
- I will acknowledge when my client has an issue that is outside my scope of knowledge and skills and recommend other resources.
- I will send a summary of each coaching session, including vision and plan for client editing (or ask the client to do so).

**Client**

- I want to improve my level of health, well-being, or performance in life or work.
- I am ready to take responsibility to make and sustain changes in at least one area.
- I am ready to invest at least three months to make improvements.
- I will be open and honest, and I will share personal information that is relevant to my health, well-being, and performance.
- I am ready to become more self-aware.
- I am curious and open to suggestions and trying new things.
- I understand that setbacks are normal on the path of change and necessary in order to establish new mindsets and behaviors.
- I will be punctual and responsive.

Whatever the language, it is recommended that the agreement established between the coach and client is in written form and revisited periodically to ensure that both parties are honoring the established boundaries and expectations. It is much easier to address concerns about the relationship based on principles which have already been agreed.

## Startup Coaching Session

An initial coaching session is typically focused on gaining a good understanding of the client's history, strengths, and goals as well as to start building a vision and plan. It is important to explain that the objectives for the first coaching session include discussing assessment results (if an assessment was part of the startup phase); learning more about the client's priorities, strengths, goals, motivators, challenges, and resources; and supporting the client in developing a plan (including a vision, three-month behavioral goals, and several first week goals). Because the initial coaching session is particularly impactful, and can cover a lot ground, it may require more time than subsequent coaching sessions, either designed as a longer initial session or divided over the course of several sessions. At their best, initial coaching sessions (Table 9.1) can range from 60 to

| **Table 9.1** | **Protocol for Designing the Coaching Relationship** |
|---|---|

**Set Expectations**

What is coaching and what is not coaching?

Introduce coach's biography.

Confidentiality and record keeping

Discuss coaching agreement principles.

Clarify expectations regarding logistics (e.g., payments, scheduling, rescheduling, and length of sessions).

Share assessment for client to complete.

**Prepare for Startup Session**

Review the well-being assessment: Seek out success, notice aliveness, consider stages of readiness, question gaps, and note concerns.

Practice mindfulness.

Remember the key coaching skills: mindful listening, open inquiry, and perceptive reflection.

Formulate curious, strengths-based inquiries.

**Session Opening**

Welcome and thank you

Thank client for completing assessments.

Review the session agenda: Confirm client's expectations and priorities, review an assessment, gather additional information, create vision, and design goals.

**Explore Well-Being Assessment**

Ask client what questions s/he has after completing the well-being assessment.

Ask client what insights s/he may have had had by completing the well-being assessment.

Gather missing information, and clarify the coach's questions.

Discuss client's medical history and need for physician release, if applicable.

90 minutes, whereas subsequent sessions can range from 20 to 60 minutes (Moore, Tschannen-Moran, & Jackson, 2002).

## Designing Visions

After coaches and clients have a good sense of each other and have developed trust and rapport, the next stage in the coaching relationship is to support the client in articulating and developing a compelling vision of his or her desired future self. Having clear goals is correlated with happiness and life satisfaction (Headey, 2008), whereas having a vision of one's best self enhances well-being and increases hope (King, 2001). A magnetic and beckoning vision contributes to the motivational energy that moves clients forward in the stages of change.

By connecting clients with a vision that considers their best experiences, core values, and generative conditions, it becomes easier for clients to imagine the way forward to a target, hence confidence grows too.

At their best, health, wellness, and life visions are as follows:

- Grounded (building on current success)
- Bold (stretching the status quo)
- Desired (what people truly want)
- Palpable (as if they were already true)
- Participatory (involving many stakeholders) (Cooperrider & Whitney, 2005)

A compelling vision identifies what people want rather than what they don't want. It's hard to see and feel the absence of something; in contrast, it's hard to ignore and resist the presence of something. This holds true for wellness and every other area of life. Wellness is not the absence of disease or the opposite of illness (World Health Organization, 2014); wellness is rather the presence of well-being and the culmination of life and health-giving practices that include mindfulness, self-compassion, energy, and all that contributes to thriving. Thriving results from tapping into one's special talents, strengths, and purpose (Benson & Scales, 2009), having a growth mindset oriented toward learning

(Dweck, 2006) and the ability to set and achieve the goals needed to grow.

Looking at wellness holistically, considering the breadth of possibility for human thriving is exciting, especially when clients have a personalized description of what they want, and believe they can do and be in the longer term (six months, one year, two years, five years, etc.). Successful coaching programs begin at this place, discovering through appreciative inquiries and reflections the values, outcomes, behaviors, motivators, strengths, and structures that clients want to realize through coaching.

Coaches avoid analyzing the causes of obstacles, barriers, setbacks, and challenges as though they were deficits to be fixed or problems to be solved. It is not helpful to ruminate for long or try to solve "why" the client has not achieved his or her dreams yet. This can generate a downward spiral of increasing discouragement and resistance. It is better to assist clients in generating new possibilities for meeting and overcoming challenges by staying positive, appreciating strengths, brainstorming alternatives, and mobilizing resources. It is empowering for clients when coaches use verbal persuasion to communicate confidence in the client's ability to move forward (Bandura, 1977).

In the early stages of change, where challenges loom large and may appear overwhelming, it's especially important to express empathy for client emotions and needs as well as express confidence that they have what it takes to succeed. This will both validate clients and reconnect them with their capacity for change and growth; it will shift the conversation in a positive direction. In the later stages of change, after clients already have a measure of self-efficacy, clients will need to brainstorm and plan action strategies, including approaches to tackle emerging challenges that will be easier to handle given the higher level of self-efficacy.

## The Importance of Motivation

As clients explore the most inspirational and feasible goals, it's important to tie those goals back to a client's reasons for change, which underlie their visions. Understanding the reasons behind the goals helps clients stay on track. For example, if a client wants to lose 10 pounds, it is important to uncover how this is connected to the vision of his or her best self (e.g., "You want to lose 10 pounds because . . . ?"). Once the reasons are pinned down, explore whether the motivator is strong enough to keep a client on track ("Is this enough to get you to the finish line? Will this reason keep you on track to make the necessary changes?"). It is important to help a client identify reasons that are strong positive motivators. Different prompts and motivators work for each client. For some, the motivator might be wanting to play with their grandchildren. In this case, posting a photo of the grandchildren on the refrigerator may help. For many, an eating log may motivate them to make conscious choices instead of eating mindlessly or in reaction to emotions. Some may want to add an avoidance motivator, such as avoiding loss of eyesight caused by diabetes. Keeping a picture of full health in mind can be a powerful motivator. Clients can breathe life into the motivator by creating a picture that they can summon later when they are making decisions between health-giving behaviors and less healthy ones.

Listen attentively for the use of words such as obstacles, barriers, setbacks, risks, or challenges. Explore what they mean by those words and what will enable them to move forward in order to achieve their goals, not just immediately but also in the long term. Staying focused on solutions and possibilities, a coach can assist clients in meeting their goals by asking questions such as:

- Tell me more about what is driving you to accomplish this goal. What is important to you about this goal? What results are you looking for?
- What have been your best experiences in accomplishing goals like this in the past?
- What values would be represented by your accomplishing this goal?
- For whom do you want to make this change?
- What structures and supports could assist you in being successful at reaching this goal?
- To what extent is this scaled appropriately with just the right amount of challenge? (Moore et al., 2002)

Although each of these topics will support the creation of a compelling vision, the importance of the client's connection to their autonomous motivation cannot be overstated (Deci & Ryan, 1985). Too often we've seen a client's first "design" of a vision being driven by external forces and validation, based on what others want of them or what they feel they "should" want for themselves. These visions aren't deeply rooted enough to plan and nourish goals that lead to sustainable action.

As clients work on their visions, the following questions can assist clients with discovering not only their long-term wishes but also with beginning to formulate their three-month goals. All of these questions will never be used with any one client on any one occasion (or the clients would feel interrogated); each of these questions add value, however, and may be useful, as clients seek to distill their vision into a provocative proposition (Tables 9.2 and 9.3).

- What would you like your health, well-being, or performance in life or work to look like in three months, one year, two years, five years, etc.?
- What do you believe is possible?
- What are the top three values in your life? How is your well-being linked to these values?
- What are the top three goals in your life? How is your well-being linked to these goals?
- What part of your life is most important to you? How does well-being fit into that?
- What would you like more of in your life? How is that linked to your well-being?
- What would you like less of in your life? How is that linked to your well-being?
- What excites you? How can we link that to your well-being?
- What motivators might enable you to overcome your inertia and start moving forward?
- What would your life be like if you achieved your vision? How would that feel?
- What would your life be like if you do not achieve your vision? How would that feel?
- What is the best-case scenario?
- What have you tried and accomplished in your life that is similar to this goal?
- What are some new possibilities that you haven't considered before?

| Table 9.2 | Protocol for Designing a Wellness Vision |
|---|---|

**Value:** Explain the value of creating a wellness vision: A vision is a compelling statement of who you are and what health-promoting, life-giving behaviors you want to do consistently.

**What's working now:** Ask about strengths and current successes: What are you currently doing to support your health and well-being? About what elements of your life do you feel best about? In what way did you contribute to making those true and/or possible?

**Strengths:** Collaborate to identify the client strengths: What are your success stories? What gives you pride? What qualities do you most appreciate about yourself?

**Thrive:** Identify ways a client can thrive: What makes you thrive? When are you most alive?

**Important:** Ask what is most important to the client right now: Given all that is going well, what are you wishing? What elements of your health and well-being do you want to improve?

**Motivation:** Discover the client's motivators: What are the benefits of making changes now? What is the driving force behind the desire to change now? What do you treasure most about potential change?

**Visualize:** Support the client in visualizing his or her vision, and describe it in detail: What are the most important elements in your vision? Tell me what your vision looks like. Paint me a picture. What would you look and feel like at your ideal level of wellness? What kind of person do you want to be when it comes to your health and well-being?

**Past successes:** Discover previous positive experiences with elements of the vision: What have been your best experiences to date with the key elements of your vision—times when you felt alive and fully engaged? Tell one or two stories in detail.

**Strengths to realize vision:** Identify the strengths and values that could be used to reach the vision: Without being modest, what do you value most about your life? What values does your wellness vision support? What strengths can you draw on to help you close that gap and realize your vision? How can the lessons from your successes in life carry over to your current situation?

**Major challenges hurting confidence:** Identify obstacles to boosting confidence: What challenges do you anticipate having to deal with on the way to reaching your vision? (Talk through multiple possibilities and express empathy.) What concerns you most?

**Strategies:** Explore the strategies and structures (people, resources, systems, and environments) needed to navigate challenges and ensure success: What people, resources, systems, and environments can you draw to help you realize your vision and meet your challenges? What strategies may be effective in helping you realize your vision and meet your challenges? (Brainstorm and clarify multiple possibilities before focusing.)

**Recap:** Reflect and summarize what you have heard the client saying about his or her vision. Collaborate on a first draft statement that captures the vision in a way that is meaningful and compelling for them.

**Commit:** Ask the client to state and commit to the vision.

| Table 9.3 | Visualization Tool for Developing a Vision |
|---|---|

This visualization exercise takes only five–10 minutes, and it can make a significant contribution, as clients seek to develop their visions.

- Close your eyes, take a deep breath from the lower stomach, and slowly breathe out. (Use this as a transition throughout the exercise.)
- In your mind, go to a quiet place where you feel comfortable, peaceful, strong, and confident. You feel relaxed. What does your quiet place look like? How do you feel being there? Notice what's around you.
- Picture yourself (one year, five years, etc.) from now. What does your health, fitness, or wellness look like? How do you look physically? What are you wearing? How does your body move? Notice any other changes in your life. Describe what you are doing, feeling, and thinking regarding your wellness.
- Imagine that it is five years from now, and you have accomplished your goals. What does it feel like? What are you doing differently? What is the same? What did you do to get there? Who's around you? What activities are you doing? Describe your health now. Who has helped you along the way?
- Think of one key word to summarize this experience and/or your commitment to health, fitness, and wellness.

Open your eyes, and let's discuss what you learned from the exercise. Debrief with a measure of confidence and an exploration of the strengths and resources clients can call on to make it so.

- What do you think is the best possible outcome of our coaching together?
- What do you think is the likely outcome of our coaching together?
- What would you like the outcome of our coaching to be? (Moore et al., 2002)

## Examples of Visions

Visions are best written in the present tense, as if they are already happening and in the client's voice. A complete vision statement might sound something like this: "I am strong, lean, and 20-pound lighter, shopping for cute, attractive new clothes for my attractive body. I am happy with lots of energy to do whatever I feel like doing. My health is better, and I am open, more patient, and social. My motivators are feeling and looking great with bountiful energy. I also want to be around a long time for my parents, nieces, and nephews. When I face challenges, such as getting too busy, discouraged, overwhelmed, or stressed out, I pause, collect myself, and take doable steps to get back on track. Healthy eating, exercise, and handling stress well are important to me and within my grasp. Through ongoing, intentional, and realistic planning, I achieve my goals and realize my wellness vision."

Or: "My wellness vision is that I have healthy eating habits and set a good example for my children. I exercise regularly so that I am delaying aging and preserving my ability to function well in my older years. I look better and feel youthful."

Or: "I have plenty of strength and stamina so that I can play energetically with my grandchildren. I am in charge of my health and feel greater well-being and contentment. I am a non-smoker (for good) and enjoy life to the fullest."

However, there is no one right way to craft a vision. Although many clients tend to choose a standard structure paragraph, some may resonate with acronyms or bullet points. For example:

- **S**table
- **T**rue to self
- **R**esilient
- **O**ptimistic
- **N**urtured by nature
- **G**rateful

And some even prefer to craft visions through creative methods such as music, poetry, and art (Moore et al., 2002).

The bottom line is that the more clients connect with their values and motivators and feel that they "own" the vision, the more successful they will be in casting a vision that compels them to take and maintain action.

## Making Visions Real: Designing Behavioral Goals

Compelling visions incorporate not only the desired outcomes but also the behaviors needed to achieve that outcome. When clients begin a coaching relationship, they typically know more about what they want (the outcomes) than about how they are going to get there (the behaviors). For example, they may say their goals are to maintain a healthy weight, increase their sense of calm, or exercise with gusto. These are outcome goals and they have their place, especially in the context of the vision statements. They reflect feelings, needs, values, and desires that can motivate and sustain behavior change. In and of themselves, however, outcome goals lead to behavior change when supported by a clear and compelling plan (Locke & Latham, 2002).

Without a clear plan, motivation alone does not propel clients into action, and it often withers in the face of adversity. With a clear plan, however, clients know what to do in order to achieve their desired outcomes and to make their visions a reality. What clients need is both willpower and waypower (Snyder, 2003).

Clear plans include behavioral goals which:

- Encourage the client to take on a *challenge* that stretches them while meeting their potential skills and abilities
- Enable clients to think about and identify the *specific actions* and behaviors they want to do next in working toward their vision, answering the question, "Now what?" (Miller, 2009)
- Encourage clients to *measure progress* against their initial baseline behaviors, adjusting and redesigning along the way. Trial and correction,

not trial and error, represents the coaching framework for action planning.

- Are grounded in the client's *motivation,* rooted in his or her values, strengths, and desires
- Support *self-efficacy and self-determination,* providing opportunities to build competence and create connection (Deci & Ryan, 2002)
- Enable coaches to measure success. Having *evidence-based data* is critical for establishing efficacy as well as credibility, not only in one's coaching practice but also in the consumer and healthcare communities (Grant, 2005).

## Is It SMART?

One formula to ensure that experiments are behavioral goals is the SMART acronym (Doran, 1981):

- **S**pecific
- **M**easurable
- **A**ction-based
- **R**ealistic
- **T**ime-bound

Assisting clients with being *specific* about the actions and behaviors in which they will engage to reach their visions will increase their levels of success. Being specific about the details of how and when is crucial because it gives clients a *time frame* in which to accomplish the goal. (It is the difference between putting something on your schedule now versus "getting around to it" when there is time.) Creating *measurable* goals identifies when success is attained.

Break down the vision into *actions* or *behaviors* that clients want to be doing on a consistent basis in three months. Each week with the client, co-construct new incremental experiment steps that will assist him or her with moving closer and closer to the three-month goals. Remind clients early and often that gradual change leads to permanent change.

*Realistic* goal setting is essential to client success. If the goal is realistic, success will follow. Quick wins and victories are important. Being successful at achieving one goal helps clients move forward with other goals. Success builds self-efficacy and self-esteem. Nothing hinders the change process more than setting unrealistic and unachievable goals.

## Why Set Goals?

Writers Locke and Latham (2002) have thoroughly researched the concept of goal setting over the course of many decades. To summarize a small section of their opus, "Building a Practically Useful Theory of Goal Setting and Task Motivation: A 35-Year Odyssey": Goals affect performance through four mechanisms. First, goals serve a directive function; they direct attention and effort toward goal-relevant activities and away from goal-irrelevant activities. Second, goals have an energizing function. High-level goals lead to greater effort than do low-level goals. Third, goals affect persistence. When participants are allowed to control the time they spend on a task, hard goals prolong effort (LaPorte & Nath, 1976). Fourth, goals affect action indirectly by leading to the arousal, discovery, and/or use of task-relevant knowledge and strategies (Locke & Latham, 1990).

"Happiness requires having clear-cut goals in life that give us a sense of purpose and direction" (Miller, 2009). Even better, when a client has success with one goal, it raises self-efficacy and increases the potential for success in other areas.

However, as indicated in the Transtheoretical Model of Change, behavioral goals must be tailored to a person's stage of change. Moving too quickly into action planning, particularly with clients in the early stages of change, will ultimately prove counterproductive. Until clients are ready, willing, and able to take action, it is important for coaches to stay in listening and inquiry mode and to assist clients with developing "thinking about," "feeling about," and/or "learning about" goals that will increase their readiness to change in a particular area. Examples of such goals drawn from the Transtheoretical Model (Prochaska, Norcross, & DiClemente, 1995), appreciative inquiry (Cooperrider & Whitney, 2005), and motivational interviewing (Miller & Rollnick, 2012) include:

- Remembering the best experiences one has had with health and wellness
- Identifying the core values that govern one's life
- Noticing one's energy in different environments
- Thinking about and writing down the components of a wellness vision

- Learning about the things that improve health and wellness.
- Weighing the pros and cons of change versus staying the same
- Thinking about the importance of making a change
- Imagining what it would feel like to be in perfect health

## Intermediate Behavioral Goals: The First Step in the Vision Quest

After a compelling vision has been articulated by your client or deferred until later, encourage the client to set goals that bring the vision closer to reality. The Wellcoaches training program encourages three-month goals as an intermediate step because it is long enough to make meaningful progress, establish some new habits, and experience the benefits, while short enough to stimulate a sense of urgency.

When working with clients to define their intermediate goals, the coach asks the client what they want to be doing consistently three (or one or two) months from now in each of the physical or mental wellness areas they included in their vision. Specific, manageable behavioral goals should be linked directly to a client's vision. For example, if clients want to be fit and trim, ask what behaviors they want to be doing consistently that will enable them to achieve that outcome.

It is important to prioritize the goal areas by importance to the client, asking what matters most and why. Then, the coach and client can brainstorm and commit to specific three-month behavioral goals in the priority areas that will help them realize the vision. Before moving on to the action plan and experimental goals, clients should clearly state and summarize their goals as part of the process of verbal persuasion (Bandura, 1977).

## Examples of Three-Month Behavioral Goals That Support Desired Outcomes

*Desired Outcome:* Improve cardiovascular health so that I live a long, active life.

| Table 9.4 | Design Three-Month Experiments/Goals |
|---|---|

| |
|---|
| Explain the nature and value of setting three-month goals. |
| Brainstorm actions that would lead to the achievement of the wellness vision. |
| Ask the client to choose three of the actions that are most important to pursue. |
| Confirm the connection of the actions to the wellness vision. |
| Assist the client in translating the actions into SMART behavioral goals. |

*Three-Month Behavioral Goal:* I will do three 30-minute walking sessions each week, at 60%–70% of my maximal heart rate with my friend Jane (Table 9.4).

*Desired Outcome:* I will increase bone density so that I am strong enough to hike the Appalachian Trail for my 70th birthday.

*Three-Month Behavioral Goal:* I will do two 20-minute strength-training sessions per week at the gym.

*Desired Outcome:* I will have peace of mind and stop taking blood pressure medicine.

*Three-Month Behavioral Goal:* I will write in my journal each evening three things that happened that day for which I am grateful and share them with my wife.

## Designing Weekly Experiments

Start the discussion of the first action plan by focusing on the intermediate goals of highest priority, then work through other areas that are important to the client. For each area, the coach will ask clients what they want to do immediately, during the next week. Weekly goals enable clients to take small manageable steps toward their longer term goals. Achieving these stepping stones is often a breakthrough in building a client's confidence.

When it comes to weekly goals, being specific about the details of how and when is crucial because it helps clients pin down the details needed to accomplish the goal. Having a mastery experience with one goal builds a sense of efficacy and helps clients be more ready, willing, and able to move forward with other goals. Nothing hinders the change process more than setting unrealistic, unachievable goals. And "low goals," as Locke and Latham (2002) call them, goals without enough challenge, produce low productivity and results.

Clients experience flow when their goals are challenging slightly beyond their skills and experience. That's the zone for clients to enter as often as possible while working on their goals. This zone is that place which is neither too hard nor too easy but rather perfectly suited for client learning, growth, and success. Because client potential is often greater than the client recognizes, don't be afraid to consider goals to which clients may exclaim, "No way!" Clients appreciate being called to go beyond what they're imagining. To assist clients with moving into this zone more frequently, the coach will encourage them to not use the words "try," "may," or "maybe." It's better to get clients to speak confidently of what they *will* do, even to the point of framing behavioral goals in the present tense, as if they were already fully true. This can positively shape client self-image and goal accomplishment (Tables 9.5 and 9.6) (Moore et al., 2002).

In addition to ensuring that goals are challenging, specific, measurable, and motivating, goals should:

- *Consider what is needed to support success.* Address environmental factors, including the client's support team and other systems that impact their successful implementation.

| Table 9.5 | Design First Experiment/ Goals |
|---|---|

| Ask the client to choose a goal that is important. |
|---|
| Explore the structures (people, resources, systems, and environments) needed to ensure. |
| Assist the client in designing a SMART behavioral goal. |
| Use a confidence ruler to improve the client's confidence in reaching the goal. |
| Ask the client to restate the goal. |
| Affirm the client's ability to achieve the goal. |

- *Have client measure confidence.* It is valuable to assess a client's confidence in his or her ability to meet a goal by asking, "What is your confidence level on a scale of 0–10 for achieving this goal?" Explore why the client did not pick a lower number or what it would take to generate a higher number. If confidence is not high enough to support success, reevaluate the goal, and make changes, and design strategies so that clients will feel confident in their ability to achieve it.
- *Measure goal importance.* To assess if clients are ready, willing, and able to change, it is essential to determine how important a goal is to them. Ask "How would you rate the importance of this goal on a scale of 0–10?" Explore why they did not pick a lower number and what it would take to generate a higher number. If clients are not ready for change, express empathy and acceptance, and explore the conditions that would generate readiness so that they recognize them when they arrive.

## The Role of Brainstorming in Goal Setting

Brainstorming, the generation of possibilities without censor, is an essential coaching skill and a fundamental part of generative moments in coaching. It is a time for coaches and clients to co-generate a wide variety of possible goals for consideration. For brainstorming sessions to be most effective, it's important to:

- Clarify the topic
- Clarify the output (what's being generated)
- Defer judgment
- Encourage bold, even wild ideas
- Build on what others say
- Be visual and specific
- Go for quantity
- Do it fast

Brainstorming enables clients to develop creative approaches and their best plans before implementation. After multiple possibilities are generated, clients can explore each one in order to determine

| Table 9.6 | Examples of Goals |
|---|---|
| **Goals That Are Not Written as Behavioral Goals** | **Behavioral Goals (Three-Month and Weekly)** |
| Do more cardiovascular exercise at the gym | Walk on the treadmill for 20 minutes at a minimum heart rate of 70% on Monday, Wednesday, and Friday after work |
| Food shopping to prepare healthier snacks | I will go to the grocery store on Saturday morning to purchase apples and almonds to have each work day. |
| I will be less stressed. | I will take an afternoon tea break each workday at 3 p.m. |
| Be more aware of how much sugar I eat | After dinner, each day this week, I will list sugary snack(s) I had throughout the day. |
| I want to be calm and more aware. | I will meditate on Saturday morning from 8:00 to 8:30 a.m. |
| I will increase my water intake and drink more water mid-morning and mid-afternoon. | I will increase my water intake from two glasses to four glasses a day by drinking an 8-oz glass of water mid-morning and mid-afternoon, Monday through Friday. |
| I will eat fewer desserts this weekend. | I will eat dessert one time this week on Saturday night and savor it slowly. |
| I will listen to music more. | I will listen to my favorite jazz album for 45 minutes on Friday evening. |
| I will do a strength-training routine of five exercises using 8-lb dumbbells. | I will do a strength-training routine of five exercises on Tuesday at 6:30 a.m. and Saturday at 10 a.m. using 8-lb dumbbells with 12 reps, with a 15-second rest between each set. |
| I will lose one pound this week. | I will eat one cup of low-sugar, high fiber cereal for breakfast from Monday through Friday. |
| I will think about what motivates me. | Before my next coaching session, I will write down my top three motivators for change and e-mail them to my coach. |
| I will make a list of the pros and cons. | I will make a list of the pros and cons for losing weight on Tuesday night before I go to bed. |
| I will pay attention to how I feel when I eat. | I will log my thoughts and emotions when I eat lunch and dinner on Tuesday and Thursday this week. |

which are the most inspirational and feasible. Most importantly, the tone of the brainstorming conversation should be positive, demonstrating high-regard for the client's creativity and capabilities, as positivity leads to enhanced problem solving and insight (Subramaniam, Kounios, Parrish, & Jung-Beeman, 2009).

## The Client Is in the Driver's Seat

Be sure clients understand that they may turn away from any challenge or goal. It is always their choice. If they seem intrigued by a behavioral goal but intimidated by the challenge, encourage them to

make a counterproposal that is more comfortable. The job of the coach is to find the balance between challenging clients to do more than they think they can do while encouraging a scaling back of goals that are out of reach. Perceptive listening is a great strategy to use in this situation and with goal setting in general. It will often promote pro-change talk, explore ambivalence, and set the groundwork to obtain a commitment.

Another way to unleash the client's ability is to encourage him or her to have self-compassion through the process of goal setting. And, one pathway to self-compassion is changing perspectives about goals by thinking of them as "experiments."

Using the design thinking premise of experimentation, viewing goals as experiments to be tested and adjusted as needed allows clients to be more likely to be resilient through the challenges of trying new behaviors and skills.

## Tracking and Measuring Outcomes Progress

Self-regulation theory (MacKenzie, Mezo, & Francis, 2012) suggests that ability to monitor oneself is a key factor in goal achievement, whereas the use of tools (such as assessments) support autonomy, a key component in self-determination theory. Therefore, it is important not only to elicit qualitative feedback regarding client progress but also to track outcomes delivered by establishing new behaviors in objective, measurable terms. When setting goals, a variety of baseline measurements and tracking techniques can be used to:

- Assist clients in tracking progress over time on selected outcomes (e.g., reduced weight or inches lost, improved life balance, better peace of mind, increased fitness, etc.)
- Help clients stay motivated toward achieving their goals
- Provide important group outcomes for a coaching practice and for the field of coaching as a whole

A combination of several tracking approaches is best because, in a given period, one measure may change, whereas another may not. Clients will be more motivated if they see positive changes in at least one behavior area through behavioral tracking.

## COACHING CASE

**Coach Carl:** "You've come up with several goal ideas that are entirely possible for you to achieve. Great work! Let's talk about how these might translate into action. Which of these do you think would be most beneficial to actually experiment with next week?"

**Wendy Well:** "You know, it may seem so simple, but the idea of taking a shower after work really sounds good."

**Coach Carl:** "What about that appeals to you?"

**Wendy Well:** "There's something about the water, the way it blocks out the sounds of the house, and it makes you feel so fresh."

**Coach Carl:** "Sounds like it calms you too."

**Wendy Well:** "Yes, there is almost nothing better than those first few minutes in the shower when the water feels hot, and you have finally gotten some time to yourself."

**Coach Carl:** "Let's take a minute and picture the evening when you come home and go straight to the shower before doing anything else. What else happens to enable you to do that?"

**Wendy Well:** "Well the kids would have to be told—well, pretty much threatened—to leave Mommy alone for a few minutes."

**Coach Carl:** "OK."

**Wendy Well:** "Actually, they are very sweet and helpful. I'm sure if I told them what I was doing they would try their best not to disturb me."

**Coach Carl:** "Sounds like you have raised respectful, loving children."

**Wendy Well:** "Thank you. I guess I would also need to tell my husband about my plan. He usually calls on his way home from work. And, I am usually in the middle of making dinner so he would have to wait to connect."

**Coach Carl:** "So, to make this happen, you would need to inform your family about what you're going to be doing and set expectations."

**Wendy Well:** "Yes, I think that's all."

**Coach Carl:** "Let's talk about how this would sound as a specific goal. We've been doing this for a few
*(continued on next page)*

weeks now. How would you phrase the goal to be specific?"

**Wendy Well:** "OK, I will take a shower when I get home from work."

**Coach Carl:** "How many days a week do you imagine yourself doing this?"

**Wendy Well:** "Let's start with Monday and Friday right after work."

**Coach Carl:** "And would you like to include what you mentioned about your family in phrasing this goal?"

**Wendy Well:** "Yes, I'll do that tomorrow."

**Coach Carl:** "Wonderful! And on a scale of 1–10, how confident are you that you'll be successful with this goal?"

**Wendy Well:** "I'd say an 8."

**Coach Carl:** "Awesome. What makes you say an 8?"

**Wendy Well:** "The image is just so fresh in my mind. I can remember how good it used to feel to have this habit, and I'm hoping it will have the same result now, 15 years later."

**Coach Carl:** "It's such a strong memory that you can almost put yourself there and believe you can do it again; that's great. I'm sure you can too. Let's talk about your other goal for next week. What goal would you like to set?"

**Wendy Well:** "I definitely want to get on the treadmill two days next week."

**Coach Carl:** "OK, so which days would you like?"

**Wendy Well:** "I'd say Monday and Friday."

**Coach Carl:** "And for how long?"

**Wendy Well:** "Let's stick with 15 minutes."

**Coach Carl:** "OK, so you will walk on the treadmill for 15 minutes Monday and Friday. And what time would you like to do it?"

**Wendy Well:** "Well I think my challenge was my tiredness during the evening time, so I want to try the morning."

**Coach Carl:** "You want to do morning, especially because you had some success with that last week?"

**Wendy Well:** "Yes."

**Coach Carl:** "And what time would you like?"

**Wendy Well:** "6:30 a.m."

**Coach Carl:** "6:30 a.m. on Monday and Friday morning."

**Wendy Well:** "Yes."

**Coach Carl:** "And how confident are you in achieving that goal?"

**Wendy Well:** "I'd say a 6–7."

**Coach Carl:** "That's a great start—more than 50% confident. What stands between you and a confidence level of an 8?"

**Wendy Well:** "It's just that 6:30 a.m. is pretty early. I know I'm going to have to really talk myself into getting out of bed."

**Coach Carl:** "What would make it easier to talk yourself into getting out of bed?"

**Wendy Well:** "I need to be sure I'm not so tired to begin with. I think trying to get to bed at a more reasonable hour during the week, at least by 10 p.m., would help."

**Coach Carl:** "So, if you got at least eight hours of sleep, you believe you would be able to get up earlier in the morning on Monday and Friday to exercise?"

**Wendy Well:** "Yes, yes definitely."

**Coach Carl:** "And how will you feel after you exercise two days this week?"

**Wendy Well:** "Amazing. I will be so proud of myself, and I imagine I'll have more energy."

**Coach Carl:** "What is your level of confidence now?"

**Wendy Well:** "Definitely an 8–9."

Over time, it is important to monitor which combination of tracking techniques will best assist the client in achieving success. During the initial sessions, ask the client which approaches they would prefer, and discuss which measurements they would like to track. It is best to start out agreeing on a few effective measurements and adjust measurements over time as motivation increases. Especially when clients have created mastery goals, or goals to develop or enhance success, they are more likely to take action to increase the chances of success, especially when supported by clear evidence (Halverson, 2010).

## Ask for Feedback on Coaching Sessions

Finally, it is important both for the coach's learning and the client's growth for the coach to get feedback on the coaching session before ending an initial coaching session. Asking questions, such as the following, provides valuable insight into what the client wants from the coaching experience:

"What was the most valuable part of today's session?"

"How could future coaching sessions best support your path?"

"Is there anything you'd like to change about our session?"

"What can I do differently to better serve you?"

Unless they are asked directly, clients typically do not tell you that they would like the coaching to be different.

Clients may be thrilled by the startup coaching sessions but it's best to inquire about their satisfaction in each session. The coach should continue getting feedback and fine-tuning the program. Requesting that the client convey feedback following the session, via email, is one way to encourage candor. If there are any doubts about the coaching chemistry, it is important to be courageous and address the concern. If the feeling is mutual, the client should be given full permission to seek another coach and be offered assistance with the process.

## Putting It All Together

To summarize, coaches help clients design compelling and engaging visions to inspire motivation and then translate their visions into realistic behavioral action steps to improve self-efficacy, increase potential for success, and learn a key life skill—developing and implementing plans to improve health and well-being.

### References

Bandura, A. (1977). Self-efficacy: Toward a unifying theory of behavioral change. *Psychological Review, 84*(2), 191–215.

Baumeister, T., & Leary, M. (1995). The need to belong: Desire for interpersonal attachments as a fundamental human motivation. *American Psychological Association, 117*(3), 497–529.

Benson, P. L., & Scales, P. C. (2009). The definition and preliminary measurement of thriving in adolescence. *Journal of Positive Psychology, 4*(1), 85–104.

Brown, T. (2008). Design thinking. *Harvard Business Review, 86*(6), 84–92, 141.

Cooperrider, D., & Whitney, D. (2005). *Appreciative inquiry: A positive revolution of change.* Oakland, CA: Berrett-Koehler.

Csikszentmihalyi, M. (1990). *Flow.* New York: Harper & Row.

Deci, E., & Ryan, R. (1985). *Intrinsic motivation and self-determination in human behavior.* New York: Plenum Press.

Deci, E. D., & Ryan, R. M. (2002). *Handbook of self-determination research.* New York: University of Rochester Press.

Doran, G. T. (1981). There's a S.M.A.R.T. way to write management's goals and objectives. *Management Review, 70*(11), 35–36.

Dweck, C. (2006). *Mindset: The new psychology* of success. New York: Random House.

Grant, A. M. (2005). What is evidence-based executive, workplace and life coaching? In M. Cavanagh, A. M. Grant, & T. Kemp (Eds.), *Evidence-based coaching: Theory, research and practice from the behavioural sciences,* 1:1–12.

Goleman, D. (1996). *Emotional intelligence: Why it can matter more than IQ.* New York: Bloomsbury Publishing.

Halverson, H. (2010). Succeed: How we can reach our goals. New York: Penguin.

Headey, B. (2008). Life goals matter to happiness. *Social Indicators Research, 86*(2), 213–231.

International Coach Federation. *Core competencies.* Retrieved March 25, 2014 from http://coach federation.org/credential/landing.cfm?Item Number=2206&navItemNumber=576

King, L. (2001). The health benefits of writing about life goals. *Personality and Social Psychology Bulletin, 27*(7), 798–807.

LaPorte, R., & Nath, R. (1976). Role of performance goals in prose learning. *Journal of Educational Psychology, 68,* 260–264.

Locke, E. A., & Latham, G. P. (1990). *A theory of goal setting and task performance.* Englewood Cliffs, NJ: Prentice Hall.

Locke, E. A., & Latham, G. P. (2002). Building a practically useful theory of goal setting and task motivation. A 35-year odyssey. *American Psychologist, 57*(9), 705–717.

MacKenzie, M., Mezo, P., & Francis, S. (2012). A conceptual framework for understanding self-regulation in adults. *New Ideas in Psychology, 30,* 155–165.

Miller, C. (2009). *Creating your best life.* New York: Sterling.

Miller, W. R., & Rollnick, S. (2012). *Motivational interviewing: Helping people change* (3rd ed.). New York: Guildford Press.

Moore, M., Tschannen-Moran, R., & Jackson, E. (2002). *First coaching session & wellness vision coaching tool.* Wellcoaches Core Coach Training Program.

Nelson, H., & Stolterman, E. (2012). *The design way: Intentional change in an unpredictable world.* Cambridge, MA: MIT Press.

Peterson, C. (2006). *A primer in positive psychology.* New York: Oxford University Press.

Prochaska, J. O., Norcross, J. C., & DiClemente, C. C. (1995). *Changing for good: A revolutionary six-stage program for overcoming bad habits and moving your life positively forward.* New York: Harper Collins.

Rosenberg, M. (2005). *Nonviolent communication: A language of life.* Encinitas, CA: PuddleDancer.

Snyder, C. (2003). *The psychology of hope.* New York: Free Press.

Subramaniam, K., Kounios, J., Parrish, T. B., & Jung-Beeman, M. (2009). A brain mechanism for facilitation of insight by positive effect. *Journal of Cognitive Neuroscience, 21*(3), 415–432.

Tschannen-Moran, M. (2004). *Trust matters: Leadership for successful schools.* Jossey-Bass.

U.S. Department of Health and Human Services. (n.d.). *Understanding health information privacy.* Retrieved December 15, 2014 from http://www.hhs.gov/ocr/privacy/hipaa/understanding/index.html

Whitworth, L., Kimsey-House, K., Kimsey-House, K., & Sandhal, P. (2007). *Co-active coaching: New skills for coaching people toward success in work and life.* Boston, MA: Nicholas Brealey Publishing.

Wolever, R., Simmons, L., Sforzo, G. A., Dill, D., Kaye, M., Bechard, E., . . . Yang, N. (2013). A systematic review of the literature on health and wellness coaching: Defining a key behavioral intervention on healthcare. *Global Advances in Health and Medicine, 2,* 38–57.

World Health Organization. (1948). *Official records of the World Health Organization  No. 2. Proceedings and final acts of the International Conference held in New York from 19 June to 22 July 1946.* Geneva, Switzerland: Author.

# CHAPTER 10

# Generative Moments

*"Whatever you can do or dream you can, begin it. Boldness has genius, power, and magic in it."*

—Goethe

## OBJECTIVES

**After reading this chapter, you will be able to:**

- Define generative moments and their value
- Discuss the source of generative moments and how to leverage these moments for significant progress
- Discuss how to use the transtheoretical model (TTM), nonviolent communication (NVC), appreciative inquiry (AI), and motivational interviewing (MI) in generative moments
- Name the skills necessary for creating and facilitating generative moments
- List the five steps in the process of creating a generative moment

## Defining the Generative Moment

Generative moments can be thought of as the peak of a coaching session. A generative moment can be filled with the high energy that comes from being ready to do something new or the peaceful calm that comes with a new way of thinking.

Generative moments occur when clients are aroused along the path of change and growth. They are the heart of coaching sessions that happen along the path to reaching or getting closer to the client's vision. In these pivotal moments, client feelings, needs, and desires are investigated around the "topic du jour." During generative moments, coaches and clients explore the nature of the agreed topic, clarify desired outcomes, brainstorm strategies, and identify next steps. In these moments, coaches and clients co-generate new perspectives and co-construct engaging designs for moving forward. Coaches often describe this collaboration as an intuitive dance.

We call these "generative" because they inspire clients to generate new ideas, perspectives, or insights. They may also uncover capacities, which can lead to bold actions that can positively alter a client's future (Bushe, 2007). Generative moments are mini transformations that energize both coach and client and catalyze the next stage of the client's progress.

As a client's emotions intensify—ranging from excited to ambivalent to fearful—coaches and clients have a unique opportunity to take risks, expand perspectives, and challenge assumptions. The more clients can discover new perspectives, capacities, and actions that will meet their needs, the more progress they will make in moving toward their visions. It's important to allow time for the generative moment in most coaching sessions in order to focus on one topic that recharges the client's batteries; this facilitates both the desire to change and the confidence to get there.

Working with a client to establish and revisit a vision can facilitate generative moments at the outset of a coaching program and whenever a session lags. It is good to revisit the vision in detail at least annually, even quarterly or monthly. Although clients commit to change and grow through building visions, lots of old and new topics emerge for consideration in coaching sessions. Many things may ignite a client's interest in a topic that calls for a generative moment—whether clients are experiencing negative or positive energy. The energy and its underlying needs make a client ripe for exploring new ways to meet those needs.

One way to think about generative moments is that they emerge as things that clients want less of (aversive indicators), things that clients want more of (attractive indicators), or some combination of the two. The former are generally accompanied by increased resistance, whereas the latter by increased readiness to pursue transformational change.

Table 10.1 provides a partial list of emotional indicators that may suggest that the client is presenting a topic for a generative moment.

Sometimes, generative moments emerge when clients are still considering change—for example, when they are in the precontemplation or contemplation stages around a particular behavior. This often happens in response to external events. Pain and bad news get people's attention, such as the message of "change or die" from a doctor. Hope and good news also have a way of getting people's attention. For example, many women stop smoking the instant they learn they are pregnant. The desire for a healthy baby eclipses the craving to smoke. At times such as these, coaches and clients have a unique opportunity to shake things up and move things forward.

## When Do Generative Moments Occur Within Coaching Sessions?

Coaching sessions tend to have a distinct beginning, middle, and end. The beginning is the warm-up phase, which is about establishing connection,

| Table 10.1 | Emotional Indicators for Generative Moments |
| --- | --- |
| **Aversive Indicators** | **Attractive Indicators** |
| Apathy, lethargy | Focus, energy |
| Worry, fear | Confidence, control |
| Anxiety | Contentment |
| Distress | Eustress |
| Boredom | Arousal |
| Sad, depressed | Happy, exhilarated |
| Unsure, hesitant | Certain, willing |
| Confused, inarticulate | Clear, articulate |
| Insecure | Safe |
| Blocked | Released |
| Stuck in the muck | Free to move |
| Out of balance | Equilibrium |
| Distracted, disengaged | Mindful, engaged |
| Rigid or loose commitment | Playful determination |
| Self-sabotage | Self-support |
| Intransigent habits | Experimental action |

exploring and appreciating recent events and experience around client goals, and clarifying the topic on which the client would like to focus. The end is about identifying goals and developing innovative strategies that will carry the client forward until the next coaching session (and beyond). The end can be considered a cool-down phase after some more energetic work in the middle. In between lies the space for the generative moment—the energetic epicenter or workout of the session. *One caveat:* Although there is a specific place and time in the process of a coaching session for the "generative moment," generativity is not limited to this time and place. Ideally, generativity is woven throughout the entire coaching session.

A good interpersonal connection and understanding of client experiences are crucial to setting in motion the first steps of the generative moment. Understanding a client's experience with his or her weekly goals, whatever the progress or lack thereof, can reveal topics around which clients have aroused energy.

Reviewing three-month goals can reconnect clients with their values, motivators, and inspiration. In the absence of judgment and in the presence of support for growth, these moments reveal what is alive in and important to clients. Encouraging clients to share stories can shed light on their feelings, their met and unmet needs, and their hopes and desires. Such is the stuff that makes for generative moments.

## What Generates Generative Moments?

Each time a client participates in a coaching session, what is important to him or her shows up for the session as well, although a warmup phase may be required to uncover what that is. To use the language of NVC, clients show up for coaching with something that is "alive" or stirring within them at that moment. It's the coach's job to listen mindfully for that life force, reflect it back to the client, and inquire about where the client wants to go with that energy (Rosenberg, 2005).

Client-driven generative moments represent a shift from traditional health education and the expert approach to change. It is not up to the coach to generate the moment. It is up to the client to show up with the energy to explore and the desire to learn. The client has that responsibility in every coaching session. Coaches enable clients to move forward positively by following the client's lead, paying careful attention to the client's feelings, needs, and desires through the use of empathy, AI, and reflections. Like a midwife supporting a mother through the transitional stages to delivery, it is not the coach's job to have "the moment" but rather to support clients through the flow of the generative moment.

Once a generative moment has run its course, coaching sessions flow easily into design and planning through the use of behavioral goals and action plans. Clients often require assistance to frame such plans as starting points for experimentation, discovery, and learning rather than as blueprints for execution. Static planning models (i.e., make the plan, implement the plan) do not reflect the dynamic of human development. Innovative planning models that include client-centered empathetic design empower clients to make realtime adjustments and improvisations, thus better supporting the client's confidence in being successful.

## Generative Moments Engage Every Coaching Skill

In order to leverage the full potential of generative moments, a coach needs to use *every* coaching skill and tool dynamically in the moment. At their best, generative moments spark the intuitive dance of coaching. Handled poorly, generative moments are not only squandered but also can set clients back in both motivation and action. The following coaching skills, introduced in previous chapters, all need to be fully engaged to effectively move clients through generative moments.

### Radiating Compassion

Generative moments require a judgment-free environment, characterized by trust and the "willingness to be vulnerable to another based on the confidence that the other is benevolent, honest, open, reliable, and competent" (Tschannen-Moran, 2004). Safety and a strong sense of support are preconditions for success in all coaching sessions. This creates optimal conditions for generative moments in which clients are challenged to stretch to the edge of their abilities. Establishing such a compassionate environment enables clients to be open and authentic so that the important stuff can get said and considered.

### Expressing Empathy

Defined as the "respectful understanding of another person's experience," empathy uses both emotional and cognitive awareness to connect with and give voice to what clients are feeling, needing, and desiring. Without receiving empathy, clients will often fail to move through and derive full benefits from generative moments. Empathy differs from pity and sympathy in that it is a coach's reflection of the client's perceived experience rather than a sharing in it. Clients are aware of empathy and presence not just consciously but also unconsciously, perhaps through the influence of mirror neurons. the influence of mirror neurons. When a coach—especially one who has developed a place of importance to the client—expresses discontent, it can send the client into physical frenzy, increasing heart rates and spreading negative energy all around (Goleman & Boyatzis, 2008).

## Mindful Listening

Defined as the "nonjudgmental awareness of what is happening in the present moment," mindfulness is a way to break free from being on autopilot. There's no way to identify generative moments apart from mindful listening. By paying attention without judgment to what's happening in oneself and in the client, coaches can help clients gain awareness of needs and choices. This is an essential component of the coaching presence required to maintain a trust-building and growth-promoting relationship.

## Evocative Inquiry

If coaches ask too many leading questions with implied "right" answers, the generative moment can be lost. True inquiry comes from the framework of "not assuming," "not knowing" the answers, and having a beginner's mind. The more coaches navigate with open-minded curiosity, especially with regard to clients' capacities and strengths, the more clients will discover about themselves and where they want to go. When coaches linger in the discovery phase of AI, with engaging questions that connect clients to their own best selves, clients are better able to put their strengths to work. "Without curiosity, we are unable to sustain our attention, we avoid risks, we abort challenging tasks, we compromise our intellectual development, we fail to achieve competencies and strengths, we limit our ability to form relationships with other people, and essentially stagnate" (Kashdan, 2009).

## Open-Ended Inquiry

When it comes to generative moments, inquiry that evokes stories and images has far more power to generate an upward spiral than does inquiry that leads to short or analytic answers. Open-ended inquiries that start with "what" or "how" are the keys to evoking such responses. Too many close-ended questions that require short "yes" or "no" answers tend to shut down this dynamic. "Why" questions can feel judgmental or can lead to analysis paralysis. Full engagement follows most directly by encouraging clients to remember and fully verbalize the stories and images of their own best selves.

## Perceptive Reflections

Asking the client too many questions in a row, even great questions, can feel like interrogation to the client and can then compromise a generative moment. Such inquiry often has more to do with the coach's desire to propel clients forward than with clients' desire to figure things out for themselves. The five forms of reflections used in MI that are especially useful in the context of generative moments are simple, amplified, double-sided, shifted-focus, and empathy reflections. They communicate the full engagement of the coach and connect the client with the motivation to change.

## Honoring Silence

In response to empathy, inquiry, and reflections, clients need to pause to think, feel, or connect with their truths. This especially happens during generative moments. It is essential for coaches to honor this silence, be comfortable with pauses, and not intrude prematurely. Once the ball is in the client's court, it is usually best to wait until the client hits it back. Intervening too quickly prevents clients from maximizing their discoveries. Silence affirms the coach's desire to hear what the client has to say and, even better, implies "I trust in your thoughts and ideas." It is a special gift to be with clients in silence, especially those who are introverted, because silence gives them time to organize their thoughts, feelings, and desires before translating them into words.

## Creative Brainstorming

Brainstorming is an essential skill of coaching, especially when it comes to generative moments. With increased motivation to change comes increased interest in specific change strategies. Such strategies are not handed to clients by coaches; rather, they are co-constructed with clients through the creative brainstorming of ideas, questions, approaches, and frameworks. Coaches and clients can generate an enormous number of possibilities without evaluating the relative merits until later. The mood can be alternately playful, insightful, courageous, and realistic. Taking turns in coming up with possibilities is a good way to build and maintain momentum through the brainstorming process.

## Unfailing Affirmation

Unfailing affirmation is about steadfastly acknowledging the client's capacities, characteristics, and strengths for change. In this way, coaches positively impact both client efficacy and self-compassion. "My certainty is greater than your doubt" expresses the framework that coaches come from in working with generative moments. When clients know that coaches believe in their capacities to change and achieve desired outcomes, they are more likely to get out of their own ways and try new strategies. Such an endorsement enables clients not only to get excited about the possibilities generated through brainstorming but also to move forward with one or more of them.

Generative moments grow out of the connection that coaches make with clients at the beginning of each coaching conversation. By establishing a "no-fault zone" where clients can blamelessly and shamelessly open up and share, coaches make it possible for clients to learn from their experiences and to move forward. Early and effective use of empathy, inquiry, and reflections in reviewing client goals (both weekly and three-month goals) helps to uncover the topics clients want to explore in greater depth.

## Facilitating Generative Moments

When creating a specific placeholder for the generative moment within the coaching session, the process includes eight primary stages:

1. Collaborates with the client to identify the topic on which to work, where he or she has aroused emotional energy and interest
2. Asks for permission to explore and work on the topic now
3. Encourages the client to describe what he or she really wants now in relation to the topic
4. Explores the strengths or values the client can leverage to move forward
5. Explores the environments the client can leverage to move forward
6. Explores decisional balance and develops discrepancy (when the client demonstrates ambivalence)
7. Engages the client in creative brainstorming of pathways forward
8. Expresses and facilitates confidence in the client's ability to move forward

## Collaborate with the Client to Identify the Topic on Which to Work Where He or She Has Aroused Emotional Energy and Interest

To identify the topic on which the client would like to focus, pay attention to the emotions, needs, desires, and values that the client has expressed throughout the session. Listen for:

- What the client is feeling
- What the client is attracted to
- What the client wants less of
- What the client is celebrating
- What needs are alive in the client
- What the client is resisting
- How ready the client is to change
- What gives the client energy
- What moves the client to action
- What the client highlights and remembers from the previous sessions

Sometimes, several topics emerge that are intertwined or are ambiguously defined. Inquiry in advance of coaching sessions (e.g., through e-mail) and the use of reflections—particularly simple reflections—are necessary to drill down to a topic underlying others or clarify a clear topic definition. Ideally, the topic of a generative moment will be self-evident to the client and coach alike. It will shine, like a light in the darkness. When that happens, it will be easy to name the topic and move to the next step.

More often, coaches and clients will float different topics for consideration until one clearly rises to the surface. Coaches may name a topic and ask if it is an area the client would like to explore. When clients agree, it may be useful to use a motivational interviewing style ruler to measure how much energy they have around that topic. If energy is low, there may be another topic worth pursuing. Or, it may be possible to invigorate a client's energy by discussing his or her energy rating.

Another approach is to engage the client's body in the search for topics. Encourage clients to pay attention to physical sensations in the moment by having them move around, strike poses, change body positions, walk, or use finger labyrinths (Rehm, 2000). Stretching, breath work, and guided meditations are also ways to invigorate the moment. Richard Strozzi Heckler (2002) refers to this as somatic coaching. The body is a resource for learning and for creating sustainable change for clients as they identify what is most important in the moment.

Alternating between open-ended inquiries and reflections is a way to clarify the topic. For example:

1. From our discussion, it sounds as though there are three potential topics which we could explore today. Here is what I have heard so far . . . (describe them succinctly)
2. We have time to work through one topic. On which one would you like to work?
3. What makes this topic the most important for our coaching today?
4. What outcome would you like at the end of today's session?

The point is not to be "right" about the best topic to pursue but rather to invite clients to look more deeply at what is alive in them. Regardless of whether the coach or client first names the topic, the key is to hold that topic as an opportunity for deeper connection and learning. The generative moment is the heart of the coaching session, and the client's heart determines the focus of the generative moment.

## COACHING CASE

**Coach Carl:** "I've watched you make such tremendous progress in the last several weeks. It's been exciting to be a part of that process, and I admire your tenacity through this. I'm excited to see you continue to take the next steps toward your three-month goals. Congratulations!"

**Wendy Well:** "Thanks. I feel good about the progress."

**Coach Carl:** "And you should savor that moment. Now, before we set goals for next week, we have a few minutes to really dive into any topic that you feel would be helpful to learn more about and understand more clearly, as you're thinking about moving toward your vision. Has anything related to your vision been on your mind that would be helpful talk through with another ear to listen?"

**Wendy Well:** "I'd like to focus on ideas for ensuring that I eat healthier. I notice that as the week goes on and I'm trying to come home from work and exercise and then I've got to get dinner, my goals kind of slide away from me, especially around eating. And my walking goal, too. At the beginning of the week, I just get on the treadmill and do it, but it seems to get harder toward the end of the week."

## Ask for Permission to Explore and Work on the Topic Now

Once a topic has been identified and clarified, the coach and client agree on the appropriateness of working on it now. Coaching always protects the freedom and choice of clients, which increases both the motivation for change and the probability of success. The client's stage of change significantly impacts both his/her readiness to address the topic as well as the approach that should be taken. If clients are in the earliest stages of change regarding a particular topic, it may be difficult for them to mount the energy necessary for a generative moment that would move them forward to action. However, in these stages, clients can do valuable thinking and feeling about possibilities, working the decisional balance for change, and exploring new supportive relationships or environments. A generative moment which builds hope can be a catalyst for increasing readiness that will eventually lead to transformational action.

## COACHING CASE

**Coach Carl:** "I'm hearing that you want to find some ways to be consistent and to be as connected to your health goals at the end of the week as you are at the beginning of the week."

**Wendy Well:** "Yes, that's it."

**Coach Carl:** "Would you like to talk about that for a few minutes?"

**Wendy Well:** "Yes, that would be helpful."

## Encourage the Client to Describe What He or She Really Wants Now in Relation to the Topic

The work of the generative moment starts with drilling down to the heart of the matter. It is a dance of self-discovery for clients, which challenges them to view and think differently about the topic and themselves. "Ah-ha!" experiences are common. Begin by tapping into or creating hope and optimism by inquiring about the client's ideal vision or optimal outcome related to the topic at hand.

Next, AI and MI models offer different paths to getting to the heart of the matter. In general, it's valuable to first start with AI to build and harvest as much positive energy and emotion as can be elicited at a given moment. Reconnection to a client's strengths and capacities may be sufficient to move forward into brainstorming and planning. MI also offers many tools to understand the roots of ambivalence, to play with ambivalence, and, even better, to resolve it. Often, coaches find themselves using a mix of both models.

## COACHING CASE Continued

**Coach Carl:** "Great! Tell me, if you could wave your magic wand, what would a week look like with consistent eating if everything just really fell in place as you wished it could."

**Wendy Well:** "It would be automatic. It would be such a routine that I just know what I'm going to bring for lunch. I would have it on hand. It would be easy to put together and I would consistently take in a lunch to work so that it would be almost every day. And, I'd feel great after lunch about what I ate. No, not just lunch—I'd feel great at the end of the day every day. No regrets."

**Coach Carl:** "And what's important about that?"

**Wendy Well:** "One, to have more energy at work and also to eat healthier so that I can do some of these things that I want to do with my life. I'd also have more time if I packed my lunch. I wouldn't have to go to the cafeteria; I could just be at my desk to eat and have quiet time. Or maybe when the weather gets nicer to go outside and sit. I think that's a nice mental break in the middle of the day. In the cafeteria, you always sit with someone, you ultimately end up talking about work again, and so you never feel like you had that break."

**Coach Carl:** "So there appear to be a number of motivators here. One is to have more energy. Another is to feel better about your choices in general. An appealing outcome of healthy eating would be having a greater sense of calm and peacefulness. Another motivator is reclaiming some down time."

## Explore the Strengths or Values the Client Can Leverage to Move Forward

It is important to approach each topic as a possibility to be explored rather than as a problem to be solved. Working from a deficit-based framework, focusing on what is wrong and what needs to be "fixed," can negatively influence how coaches view client potential and can compromise client self-efficacy.

Instead, masterful coaches explore a topic from a strengths-based perspective, even when clients are experiencing resistance to change. Strengths-based inquiries focus on what is meaningful and compelling to clients more than on what they do not want. In addition, they invite clients to recall and reconnect with past successful experiences.

The benefits of using strength-based inquiries are plentiful. They include generating hope, optimism, and other kinds of positivity; reminding clients of their capabilities; and encouraging more of the behaviors that generated previous success. Remember the AI principle: that which we appreciate appreciates. Using the AI interview protocol, the following represent a sample of questions that can generate positive shifts in thoughts and behaviors:

- Tell me about a time when you experienced a similar challenge and navigated your way through it.
- What did success feel like?
- What are the values reflected in and how you have handled this situation?
- How does this connect with your vision?
- What are the needs that would be met if this vision were realized for you?
- What are the structures (people, places, things, tools, routines) that would enable you to be successful with this goal?
- What are your hopes for how you would like to handle this issue in the future?
- Name your main wish.

The primary objective of using the AI approach first is to engage clients in conversations that reconnect to their vitality—that place of deep longing that brought them to coaching in the first place. Such questions and requests shine a light on the hope and enthusiasm clients have for their visions and realign the situations with their visions.

## Explore the Environments the Client Can Leverage to Move Forward

As Peterson and Seligman (2004) found in studying the prevalence of universal strengths and values, self-regulation is one of the least valued and used strengths. Self-regulation is vital in the

change process. It manifests in diligently planning, preparing, and executing behavioral experiments; unpacking learning; followed by adjusting the what, how, and when of practicing new behaviors, over and over again. Given that clients make behavioral decisions and choices all day long under

## COACHING CASE Continued

**Wendy Well:** "Yes. That's kind of the way it felt when I took my lunch on Monday."

**Coach Carl:** "That's powerful. Tell me about Monday. That was a clear success. What led to that success? What were the things that were going on in your life on Sunday that supported Monday's healthy eating?"

**Wendy Well:** "Well basically, Sunday is our family day. I clean, grocery shop, do errands, and domestic things on Saturday. So Sunday is just kind of a down day, and in the evening, I always take time to kind of regroup and reorganize for the week. So it's a calm evening I guess. It's not as crazy as the other evenings when you get home from work late and have so much to do."

**Coach Carl:** "You have this space on Sunday that you know you can use. It sounds like Sundays offer the opportunity to make some of those more productive things happen."

**Wendy Well:** "Right. Just in general, that's what I've always done. So it was very easy to fit the lunch in and prepare and get organized for the lunch on Sunday night because I kind of take that time to organize anyway."

**Coach Carl:** "OK, so you set aside the time. What else did you have in place on Sunday that made it easier to make this happen?"

**Wendy Well:** "I think I knew what I had in the refrigerator because I just bought it on Saturday. I knew it was fresh, I knew it was there; it was kind of more present in my mind and in my thinking, too."

**Coach Carl:** "OK got it. You had the lunch supplies you needed, you remembered what supplies you had, and you had the time to prepare lunches."

strong influences of their environments, how then can clients adjust their environments to bolster their success, including boosting of much-needed self-regulation?

First of course, the coaching process provides a valuable support to enhancing self-regulation in and of itself. Coaches can then help clients appreciate how their environments affect their self-regulation and encourage clients to consider "what might happen, when it might happen, and how it might affect" their progress. "Coaching the environment" is a proactive strategy that supports goal achievement (Gollwitzer & Sheeran, 2006). Clients can design environments that enable them to be more competent, a key psychological need and resource as we learned in exploring self-determination theory. The coach and client can together find the environments that enhance completion of new experiments, and they can design structures (people, places, things) that increase the likelihood of mastery experiences.

## Explore Decisional Balance and Develop Discrepancy (When the Client Demonstrates Ambivalence)

When the principles of AI do not uncover the heart of the matter and elevate clients' readiness to move in the directions of their desires, MI tools can be useful to help them understand and dislodge their "stuckness," resolve ambivalence, and move forward.

Expressing empathy, developing discrepancy, rolling with resistance, and supporting self-efficacy are all designed to create a safe space for clients to explore their thoughts, feelings, needs, and intentions. When the space is right, clients can leave behind their uncertainty to change and open themselves to new possibilities. This is often a critical part of successfully coaching clients through their generative moments.

Inviting clients to describe their authentic reasons for changing (change talk), instead of telling and selling clients on why they "should" change, is a challenging shift for a new coach. "Get into fishing and out of sales," says motivational interviewing trainer and psychologist Robert Rhode. Keep in mind that clients are more likely to move in the direction of positive change when they have figured out and described in their own words what outcomes they really want and clarified what challenges may be getting in the way and what it will take to reach their goals (change talk). After clients have been "sitting in the muck" for a while, struggling with the discrepancy or conflict between the needs to not change and the needs to change, they will gain motivational energy by a desire to resolve the discrepancy and get readier to take action to move forward.

Coaching tools will not work unless the coach starts with the intention of understanding the client's experience. The more coaches try to manipulate behavior or force an outcome, the more these tools will increase rather than decrease resistance. When that happens, coaches are working against rather than supporting generativity. Self-determination theory makes it clear that the human propensity for growth only happens when change is freely or autonomously chosen in the moment and supported by competence and relatedness (Markland, Ryan, Tobin, & Rollnick, 2005).

## Engage the Client in Creative Brainstorming of Pathways Forward

Once change talk has begun and client energy is higher, it's helpful to engage clients in the light-hearted generation or brainstorming of ideas and approaches for moving forward. In brainstorming, possibilities are generated but not critiqued or evaluated. A good rule is the more the better when it comes to idea generation. Coaches and clients can take turns in the generation of ideas and experiments. It can be challenging for coaches and clients to generate possibilities in the moment, but it is well worth the effort. Sometimes, coaches come up with possibilities that clients would never have thought of on their own. When coaches take a turn, clients are given the space to think more deeply about or jump off from a possibility in a whole new direction suggested by the coach. Such brainstorming is valuable and usually fun during generative moments.

It is helpful to designate a particular time during the generative moment for brainstorming ideas, questions, or approaches. Brainstorming too early can overwhelm clients and provoke resistance. However, failing to brainstorm at all can squander the potential of the moment, either because no possibilities are generated or because one possibility takes over before others are considered. Running with the first idea that comes up is not only limiting but also may be dangerous. As French philosopher

## COACHING CASE Continued

**Coach Carl:** "I'm wondering if we might take some time to generate some new ideas to make this easier for you. How can we make this goal be more consistently achievable, keeping in mind some of the things that you learned on Sunday, some of those environmental factors that really supported you in being successful? Maybe we could just generate five to seven things you might put in place throughout the week to be more successful here. Anything goes when we are brainstorming; there are no bad ideas. How does that sound?"

**Wendy Well:** "Sure, that would be helpful!"

**Coach Carl:** "OK, perhaps we can go back and forth with ideas. Do you want to throw out an idea?"

**Wendy Well:** "I guess one idea came to mind when I said I knew what I had on hand. Maybe it would be helpful to keep more of a list or something on my refrigerator. If I checked them off as I took them so I could see what was left, that might be more of a reminder of what I had."

**Coach Carl:** "OK, keeping a list on the fridge. Great. I have an idea around making a meal list on Sunday; you could plan out what your lunches will be for the rest of the week."

**Wendy Well:** "Yes, that could work."

**Coach Carl:** "What else?"

**Wendy Well:** "Maybe buying fruit at the beginning of the week and taking it to work with me."

**Coach Carl:** "OK, taking in some of the supplies, perhaps on Monday, so you have them on hand."

**Wendy Well:** "Yes. I could pack them in Monday mornings."

**Coach Carl:** "Here's another idea; every night from 6:30–6:40 a.m. can be your lunch packing time."

**Wendy Well:** "That could be, except that's my exercise time too. I guess if I could pack my lunch on the treadmill, I'd be all set."

**Coach Carl:** "Now that would be quite a feat! OK, well we'll play with how these ideas might look in the real world. Let's get one more."

**Wendy Well:** "One more. I could bring a lunch that is premade, that I don't even have to fix, like maybe salads in containers or something like that."

**Coach Carl:** "Pre-prepared lunches. OK, that would be less effort. Let's shift gears and revisit and reignite your motivation. Wendy, how important is it to you to eat healthy on a more consistent basis? And perhaps we can use that familiar ruler from 0 to 10, 10 being most important."

**Wendy Well:** "This one is an 8 or a 9. I think it is kind of a cornerstone for the other things that I want to do to be healthy and energetic. I was doing well with breakfast and dinner, but lunchtime has been getting away from me and dragging down my confidence in other areas."

**Coach Carl:** "It feels kind of like a foundation for success in other areas."

**Wendy Well:** "Yes, and I think eating a healthy lunch will improve my energy for work in the afternoon. Sometimes, eating less healthy cafeteria food makes me sleepy and wanting a nap."

**Coach Carl:** "You notice that there are good consequences when you eat a healthy lunch both for the afternoon, the whole day, and beyond."

Emile Chartier (1959) writes, "Nothing is as dangerous as an idea when it is the only one you have."

Basic protocols for successful brainstorming include the following:

- Setting a time limit
- Withholding judgment or evaluation of ideas
- Encouraging wild, fun, and exaggerated ideas
- Letting no idea go unsaid
- Setting a minimum number of ideas or questions to generate
- Building on the possibilities put forth by the other
- Combining and expanding ideas
- Asking permission to contribute ideas

With many compelling and relevant ideas in mind, the client will eagerly move with confidence and energy to designing action plans, the next step of the coaching session. With high self-efficacy, clients will be ready, willing, and able to commit to specific behaviors that will contribute to realizing their visions.

### Express and Facilitate Confidence in the Client's Ability to Move Forward

The transition to designing action plans at the end of the generative moment is made compelling when the coach champions and supports the client's ability to move forward with one or more of the new ideas or approaches. Forward movement is more appealing when clients believe they have the ability to turn the new ideas into action. Hence, coaches not only support self-efficacy throughout the entire coaching session; this is especially important as the generative moment comes to a close.

By acknowledging what clients brought to the generative moment, the good work they have done in brainstorming, and their capacity to see their dreams through to fruition, coaches enable clients to commit themselves and to take actions that will generate success.

W. H. Murray (1951) of the Scottish Himalayan expedition famously addressed this dynamic when he wrote:

> Concerning all acts of initiative (and creation), there is one elementary truth, the ignorance of which kills countless ideas and splendid plans: that the moment one definitely commits oneself, the providence moves too. All sorts of things occur to help one that would never otherwise have occurred. A whole stream of events issues from the decision, raising in one's favor all manner of unforeseen incidents, meetings and material assistance, which no one could have dreamth would have come his or her way. I learned a deep respect for one of Goethe's couplets: Whatever you can do, or dream you can, begin it. Boldness has genius, power, and magic in it. (pp. 6–7)

Championing the client at the close of the generative moment is an essential part of masterful coaching.

## Relational Flow in Generative Moments

The earlier process provides a framework for handling generative moments. Yet, in many respects, these moments are not "handled"; rather, they have a playful, surprising, improvisational, flowing quality that cannot be scripted. The best generative moments move seamlessly and organically in flow—they feel like a dance—sometimes slow, sometimes quick, or more like a salsa dance.

Given their impact, new coaches can feel pressure to demonstrate great skill, wisdom, or technique. The most important thing to remember is that generative moments are about the client's needs and desires. By following the client's lead, coaches can ease their way into collaborative, co-creative conversations. Coaches remember that they are in partnership rather than in charge, and they remain attentive to the client's energy and insights rather than distracted by their own thoughts and inspired rather than inspirational. At their best, generative moments feel intense, exciting, deep, powerful, and moving, but not hard. Generative moments flow.

### What Is Relational Flow?

Relational flow, another way to define generative moments, happens when coaches and clients perceive themselves as being in sync and engaged in generative, interdependent, collaborative dialogue. In reflecting on peak coaching experiences, coaches and clients often describe their best moments as like being in an intuitive dance: "a relational dynamic between coaches and clients when they enter a zone where they are fully challenged at a high level of skill and awareness. This dynamic, conceptualized as 'relational flow,' may underpin how and when both coaches and clients make large steps forward in their work" (Moore, Drake, Tschannen-Moran, Campone, & Kauffman, 2005).

It is a challenge to create relational flow, let alone capture or measure it. That's because it is an intuitive and synergistic dynamic that is created by the coach, the client, and the field *between* the two. Like learning to dance, the fundamental steps must be mastered before style, fluidity, and flow can be demonstrated. In flow, coaches aren't married to a plan that determines what happens next or attached to a particular outcome. Instead, they are able to use what is happening in the moment to determine what will happen in the next moment, improvising with agility based on what is most important to the client in the present moment.

## What Supports Relational Flow?

Although research into the dynamic continues, several bodies of knowledge illuminate and support the intuitive dance of coaching. These include the following:

- *Flow studies*—As defined by Mihaly Csikszentmihalyi (2000), flow exists when one is engaged in a challenging situation that requires fully engaging and stretching one's skills at a high level in response. In flow, one becomes immersed in an activity with greater attention, less effort, and an altered sense of time.
- *Reflective practitioner*—The ability to dance effortlessly also comes from practice. A coach with experience is "less tied to explicit rules, processes, and contextual clues in order to know how to act effectively—and yet does so with less effort" (Moore et al., 2005). Experienced coaches rely more on intuitive thoughts and perceptions. They draw on previously successful experience—lots of it. The intuition of a master is powerful, whereas for novices, it's limited.
- *Readiness to change*—A client's ability to engage in flow depends on his or her stage of change.

The coach must be cognizant of the client's readiness to change and adjust the approach accordingly. Masterful coaches do not push clients through the stages of change; rather, they draw clients out by honoring the needs of the moment.
- *Emotional intelligence*—As defined by Daniel Goleman (1998), emotional intelligence is the ability to "recognize our own feelings and those of others, for motivating ourselves, and for managing emotions well in ourselves and in our relationships." In the coaching conversation, the competencies that contribute to emotional intelligence are necessary for intuition and use it for positive outcomes; this is an essential part of the empathy that contributes to relational flow.
- *Relational competence*—In the generative moment, the dance is a collaboration between two connected people. From relational cultural theory (Jordan, Walker, & Hartling, 2004; Walker & Rosen, 2004), we know that growth through connection, rather than separation, leads to healthy functioning. In deep connection with their coaches, clients feel more vital, empowered, clear, worthy, and driven toward more connection with others (Moore et al., 2005).

Hall and Duvall (2005) conclude:

The coach dances with a client to facilitate the unleashing of potentials and the experience of change. The dialogue dance creates motivation and energy in the player or the client. The dance creates readiness for change, the power to change, and the leverage for change. In this dance, new frames of mind are co-created for facilitating that change. The dialogue is a dance around support, celebration, accountability, fun, and actualizing potential. It's a dance for enabling dreams to come true. Do you want to dance? (p. 6)

## References

Bushe, G. (2007). Appreciative inquiry is not (just) about the positive. *Organization Development Practitioner, 39*(4), 30–35.

Chartier, E. (1959). *About religion*. Paris: University Press of France.

Csikszentmihalyi, M. (2000). *Beyond boredom and anxiety: Experiencing flow in work and play*. San Francisco: Jossey-Bass.

Goleman, D. (1998). *Working with emotional intelligence*. New York: Bantam Books.

Goleman, D., & Boyatzis, R. (2008). Social intelligence and the biology of leadership. *Harvard Business Review, 86*(9), 74–81.

Gollwitzer, P., & Sheeran, P. (2006). Implementation intentions and goal achievement: A meta-analysis of effects and processes. *Advances in Experimental Social Psychology, 38*, 69–119.

Hall, L. M., & Duval, M. (2005). *Meta-coaching, volume II: Coaching conversations for transformational change.* Clifton, CO: Neuro-Semantics.

Jordan, J., Walker, M., & Hartling, L. M. (2004). *The complexity of connection: Writings from the Stone Center's Jean Baker Miller Training Institute.* New York: The Guilford Press.

Kashdan, T. (2009). *Curious?: Discover the missing ingredient to a fulfilling life.* New York: HarperCollins.

Markland, D., Ryan, R. M., Tobin, V. J., & Rollnick, S. (2005). Motivational interviewing and self-determination theory. *Journal of Social and Clinical Psychology, 24*(6), 811–831.

Moore, M., Drake, D., Tschannen-Moran, B., Campone, F., & Kauffman, C. (2005). Relational flow: A theoretical model for the intuitive dance. *Proceedings of the Third International Coach Federation Coaching Research Symposium.* Lexington, KY: International Coach Federation.

Murray, W. H. (1951). *The Scottish Himalayan expedition.* London: J. M. Dent & Sons.

O'Hanlon, B., & Beadle, S. (1997). *A guide to possibility land: 51 methods for doing brief, respectful therapy.* New York: W. W. Norton.

Peterson, C., & Seligman, M. E. P. (2004). *Character strengths and virtues: A handbook and classification.* New York: Oxford University Press.

Rehm, J. (2000). Pathways to peacefulness. *On Wisconsin.* Winter, 28–32.

Rosenberg, M. S. (2005). *Nonviolent communication: A language of life.* Encinitas, CA: PuddleDancer Press.

Strozzi Heckler, R. (2002). Power of somatics. In Strozzie Institute. Retrieved April 27, 2015 from http://www.strozziinstitute.com/somatic+coaching+mastery.

Tschannen-Moran, M. (2004). *Trust matters: Leadership for successful schools.* San Francisco: Jossey-Bass.

Walker, M., & Rosen, W. (2004). *How connections heal: Stories from relational-cultural therapy.* New York: Guilford Press.

# CHAPTER 11

Conducting Coaching Sessions

> *"Good fortune is what happens when opportunity meets with planning."*
>
> —Thomas Alva Edison

## OBJECTIVES

**After reading this chapter, you will be able to:**

- Identify the process for conducting coaching sessions following an evidence-based coaching model
- Follow a checklist for evidence-based coaching programs and sessions (Appendix A)

## Introduction

Among the International Coach Federation's core coaching competencies is "managing progress and accountability," enabling clients to move from Point A (where they are today) to Point B (where they want to go). There are many approaches to the design and process of coaching programs and sessions that facilitate movement to Point B.

Although there is never only one "right" way to do coaching, clients and coaches enjoy structure as a means to understand and gain mastery in the process of facilitating change. As coaches gain experience and grow their toolboxes, they can modify the process of coaching sessions in ways that maintain engagement for themselves and their clients.

Since 2002, Wellcoaches has developed, practiced, and continually refined a protocol for coaching programs and sessions, which is now evidence-based, proving highly effective in a growing number of outcomes studies. This protocol provides a valuable handrail for new coaches so that they are more effective from the outset. This coaching protocol has been applied in a variety of settings with diverse populations. A few examples include the following:

1. Polak, Dill, Abrahamson, Pojednic, and Phillips (2014)—improving consumption of healthy food in a patient with diabetes through wellness coaching
2. McGloin, Timmons, Coates, and Boore (2014)—wellness coaching for type 2 *diabetes*
3. Sforzo, Kaye, Ayers, Talbert, and Hill (2014)—wellness coaching for smoking cessation
4. Roy, Lisowski, and Roberts (2014)—wellness coaching with physician-referred patients with chronic health conditions
5. Sforzo (2013)—wellness coaching for Ithaca College employees
6. Sherman, Crocker, Dill, and Judge (2013)—at Massachusetts General Hospital (MGH), health coaching in the primary care setting for employees
7. Schwartz (2013)—wellness coaching as an alternative to bariatric surgery

8. Berna (2013)—wellness coaching in a tribal community healthcare center with patients with diabetes

9. Galantino et al. (2009)—wellness coaching for cancer survivors who had significant improvements in depression scores, exercise behaviors, and quality-of-life scores

Having introduced the coaching session protocol for designing the relationship, a vision, and three-month behavioral goals in Chapter 9, the focus of this chapter is on the protocol for ongoing coaching sessions that follow the startup coaching sessions. Appendix A has a coaching program checklist for four phases—prospect phase, startup, ongoing sessions, and program close or wrap-up.

## Prepare for a Coaching Session

The most important moment of a coaching session is arguably the minute right before it starts (Table 11.1). That's when coaches relax and clear their minds, set their intentions, and get into a coaching mindset. If growth and self-determination come from relationships, the coach must be attentive to the nurturing of that relationship at every opportunity, remembering the following:

*Confidence is contagious.* When coaches communicate their genuine confidence that clients can be successful, client confidence will also improve.

*What is appreciated appreciates.* The more the coach focuses on what clients want rather than on what they don't want, the more energy and ideas clients will have for moving forward.

*To listen for the client's needs.* The more the coach sets aside his or her own agenda in favor of listening for the client's agenda, the more clients will

| Table 11.1 | Prepare for a Session |
|---|---|
| Prepare: Review client assessment results and client communication. |
| Get present: Practice mindfulness, set intention, and connect to purpose. |
| Get curious: Consider initial strengths-based inquiries. |

discover about themselves and create new perspectives, possibilities, and learning.

*To tell the truth.* The more a coach helps clients reveal themselves to themselves through empathy, authenticity, and honesty, the more and progress clients will make more quickly. A coach can use courage and kindness to notice and reflect discrepancies between goals and current behaviors and to note downward thought patterns or downward spiral thinking.

*To trust intuition.* The more deeply the coach listens to his or her own intuition during coaching conversations, the more deeply clients will connect with their own intuition. That helps leads to the intuitive dance or the generative moments of coaching.

## Session Opening

First, let's address time management. In an ongoing coaching session, weekly, biweekly, or monthly, for example, the following percentages indicate how coaches may want to spend their time with clients. The percentages indicate the number of minutes that coaches may want to spend with clients in each section during a 30-minute session.

- Session opening—7% (two to three minutes)
- Weekly goal review—20% (five to seven minutes)
- Three-month goal review (monthly or so)—7% (two to three minutes)
- Generative moment—40% (10–12 minutes)
- Goal setting—20% (five to seven minutes)
- Session close—6% (two to three minutes)

This could be compared to a warmup, a workout, and a cool-down. For longer sessions of 40–60 minutes, more time becomes available for generative collaboration, a deeper dive into the journey of change, for example, shifting change-hindering mindsets to possibility-creating mindsets. Thinking through time management before each session and making adjustments as situations come up will assist coaches and clients alike with being more successful and satisfied with the coaching experience.

Trust and rapport are not earned once and for all during the first coaching session. They are earned all over again, each time coaches and clients meet. Understanding this phenomenon, it is important to be prepared to start the session by asking about the client's feelings and energy now in that moment and to listen mindfully to the response.

Next, explore the highlights rather than the problem areas since the last session. When clients show up with great discouragement or low energy, the focus on highlights may reconnect them with their own resourcefulness and potential. When that does not happen directly, the coach should express empathy for the client's feelings and needs. By understanding and supporting clients in these ways, coaches assist clients in rebooting and regaining their balance so they can consider anew the possibilities for change (Table 11.2).

| Table 11.2 | Session Opening |
|---|---|
| Asks how the client is right now "in this moment" |
| Uses reflections to show understanding of the client's state |
| Asks the client to share the best thing that happened from previous week(s) |
| Reflects something positive about the client (e.g., highlights, strengths, or emotions) |
| Asks client to select the first weekly goal to be discussed |

## COACHING CASE

**Session Opening**

**Coach Carl:** "Hello Wendy. How are you today?"

**Wendy Well:** "I'm fine Carl, thanks."

**Coach Carl:** "That's good to hear. I'd love to get a little more specific about what "fine" means. You remember we used an energy scale before. I'm curious about how you're feeling on a scale of 1–10, with 10 being you could climb a mountain, and 1 being you'd just like to climb under the covers. Where are you today?"

**Wendy Well:** "Late last week, I probably would have said 1 (one) because I had a business trip, and I was traveling a lot, but today I'm kind of getting back on track again, so I'd say I'm probably a 6 or a 7."

**Coach Carl:** "So you were feeling stretched by travel last week, but you're moving up the scale. And tell me what a 6 or a 7 feels like. How would you describe that?"

**Wendy Well:** "A 7 is when the alarm goes off or before the alarm goes off, you get up and get ready and feel good about getting things done. I'll throw a load of clothes in the laundry or take the dog for a walk, get things done and going even before I go to work. It just seems like I have the energy to do everything that I need and want to do."

**Coach Carl:** "You feel more productive and energetic. Traveling sometimes is tiresome, especially when there are time changes."

**Wendy Well:** "That's right, yes. Productive, that's a good word. I'm being more productive at work too. I know if I have more energy, I'm more productive at work."

**Coach Carl:** "As you think about the last week, settling back into a routine and enjoying that, you're meeting all of the goals that you've set out to meet each day. What is there to celebrate? What's been the best thing that's happened to you in the last several days?"

**Wendy Well:** "I think getting back into the exercise. I also notice that I just find myself walking more. I'll take my dog for a little bit longer of a walk, or I'll walk up to the corner and back. And I've just noticed this week that happens kind of on its own without really even trying to do it. So that's been great."

**Coach Carl:** "Wendy, that's exciting. I know when our sessions started, you were finding it hard to get motivated on some of those extra steps, and I suspected it was really in you all along. It's terrific to hear that the stretch in your exercise is just starting to happen naturally without thinking about it."

# Goal/Experiment Review

Once a connection has been reestablished, it's time for clients to select the first goal to be discussed. Don't assume that this will turn out to be the most important goal for the client. Rather, it is an opening for collaboration, an opportunity to get into the dynamic of coaching. Most clients will set two to five behavioral goals to work on between coaching sessions. Each of these goals should be reviewed to discover client accomplishments, challenges, and lessons. Building on the principles of positive psychology and appreciative inquiry (AI), it is most effective to begin with a positive "best experience" question for each goal.

When reviewing goals, it's best to start by asking about the things that went well and the lessons that were learned. Clients should first be directed to consider what they accomplished rather than start with what they did not accomplish. For example, "Unfortunately, I put butter on my whole wheat toast for breakfast four times this week" can be reframed as: "I was successful in my goal of substituting peanut butter for butter on whole grain toast for breakfast five times 20% of the time this week." By reframing goal accomplishment in positive terms and by asking positive questions, coaches help clients find the confidence and energy to move forward. Positive emotions create an upward spiral, leading to the creativity and openness needed for tackling the challenges of goals that weren't achieved so easily or goals yet to be dreamed (Fredrickson, 2009).

Examples of inquiries for the review process include the following:

- What was your best experience with your goals in the past week?
- What percentage of achievement did you reach for this goal? What contributed to this level of success?
- What kept it from being lower?
- What could have made it higher?
- What do you like about this goal?
- What did you learn from this experience?
- What challenges did you face along the way?

- Do you think this goal is too ambitious, too cautious, or just right?
- When you think about this goal, what feelings does it stimulate, and what needs does it meet?

Inquiries such as these honor the client's autonomy and competence while enabling him or her to grow in partnership with a trusted collaborator, the coach.

## Accountability in Coaching

Accountability means monitoring and giving an account of what was done, what happened, what worked, what didn't work, and what one wants to do differently in the future. When such accountability comes from the coach-client collaboration, discussing what has been accomplished in objective rather than judgmental terms, clients often become empowered to reach their goals more consistently and effectively.

When it comes to health and well-being, people are generally accountable only to themselves—and that often isn't enough, especially in the early stages of change. With such isolation and anonymity, it's easy for motivation, diligence, and follow-through to slip. Building in accountability helps ensure that clients remain on track.

Checking on a client's experience with goals is not the same as pestering or nagging. It is rather a welcome conversation that includes reviewing a client's best experiences with his or her goal design and the learning that arises from it. When appropriate, the coach can assist clients with reframing "failure talk" as "learning opportunities."

In a complete absence of judgment, exploring progress as an accountability activity is an empowering conversation that provides structure, measurement, and support without being an unpleasant experience for a client (Table 11.3). The key is to keep it light without failing to raise important topics. To be effective, it's important for coaches not to get attached to an outcome, remembering that a coach is not a client's boss or parent.

| Table 11.3 | Experiment/Goal Review |
|---|---|
| Explores full experience with weekly goal, starting with the positive |
| Uses reflections to show listening and understanding of the goal experience |
| Expands inquiry about the client's best experience with his or her weekly goal |
| Responds to client challenges with judgment-free reflections and inquiries |
| Asks what the client learned from his or her experience |
| Affirms the client's strengths, choices, and/or situation |
| Inquires about the client's percentage of success |

Taking a design perspective (Brown, 2008) once the goals (or experiments) have been tested, evaluation of their effectiveness is the next stage. It is important to explore both how clients feel about their progress as well as the factual aspects of progress.

## Three-Month Goal Check-In

It is not necessary for a client to revisit his or her vision and three-month goals every week. It is important, however, to do so at least monthly in order for the weekly experiments and goals to stay connected to a client's larger vision and purpose. It is empowering to connect the dots between smaller incremental steps and larger motivating life goals.

# COACHING CASE

*Experiment/Goal Review*

**Coach Carl:** "Which of your goals from last week would you like to discuss first?"

**Wendy Well:** "Let's talk about my walking goal first."

**Coach Carl:** "Tell me what happened with the walking goal, including those things you feel satisfied about or grateful for that are related to that goal."

**Wendy Well:** "I think I'm just so proud of myself for exercising as soon as I get home for work even though it is hard. It is so easy to go back to my computer and try to respond to a few more e-mails. But I say, "'No, I'm going to do it because I know Carl is going to be asking me about it.'" That's a big change for me."

**Coach Carl:** "That's interesting. And of course it's really not just about checking in with me. I'm curious what it was, aside from knowing you had to tell someone about it. What was it that got you on the treadmill?"

**Wendy Well:** "I think knowing how good I feel when I get off the treadmill. And it really only takes 15–20 minutes. In the past, when I would start an exercise program, it was at least 30 minutes, and so I would stop doing it; it was just too long and boring. So just knowing that it's only a short amount of

time, and then recalling how good it felt last week was energizing."

**Coach Carl:** "I just want to make sure I'm clear with what happened with that goal. I know your intention was to walk for 15 minutes on Monday and Friday at 6:30 a.m. What actually did happen for you?"

**Wendy Well:** "I did it on Monday for 15 minutes at 6:30 p.m. I don't know why I said I could do it on Friday because co-workers and I often meet for an early breakfast meeting on Friday. So as I was looking at my goals, I decided to do it on Thursday night instead."

**Coach Carl:** "That's good forethought, planning, and commitment to your goal!"

**Wendy Well:** "Yes, and part of it was that I traveled back from a work trip on Thursday, so I actually looked forward to the treadmill after being cooped up on a plane."

**Coach Carl:** "What did you most enjoy about getting the exercise in?"

**Wendy Well:** "I hate to say it, but part of it was being done with it. I mean it does feel good, but I can't say I'm one of those exercise lovers. Still, it feels good to be on track."

*(continued on next page)*

**Coach Carl:** "I hear you saying that it wasn't without challenges."

**Wendy Well:** "Yes, it takes some strong self-encouragement talk sometimes."

**Coach Carl:** "Something you are getting better at. So what's your takeaway from this experience as we're thinking about goals for next week?"

**Wendy Well:** "I guess the takeaway is to just do it and to be prepared to be flexible with it too. Instead of saying, "'Oh Friday isn't going to work'" and throwing out the whole goal, I reset and made it work."

**Coach Carl:** "I just want to affirm the way that you're being both forgiving and flexible. That mindset is really going to support you in staying positive as you move forward. So in terms of your percentages of success here, from 0% to 100%, how successful were you?"

**Wendy Well:** "I would say 100%."

**Coach Carl:** "Congratulations. And, which goal would you like to talk about next?"

**Wendy Well:** "Well, the nutrition goal. That one didn't go quite as well. I did have a good lunch on Monday but not on Wednesday or Friday."

**Coach Carl:** "OK, we will definitely explore what happened on Wednesday and Friday, so hold those thoughts for a moment. Let's focus on Monday first. Tell me about what happened on Monday."

**Wendy Well:** "I had been to the grocery store on Sunday, and we stocked up on things for lunches and other things in general. So I had fruit, and I had some of those small bags of carrots and some things that were easy to pack. On Sunday night, I do just generally make sure the house is clean and the clothes are done, so I'm ready to start the week being very productive. I had laid out a few things that didn't need to be refrigerated, and they were there and ready to go and Monday morning when I got up, so it was very easy to put together and take with me."

**Coach Carl:** "It was part of your routine, and you also had some convenience built into that routine, because you had some of the things on hand that you needed."

**Wendy Well:** "Right."

**Coach Carl:** "And how did you feel on Monday when you accomplished that goal as you were eating that healthy lunch?"

**Wendy Well:** "It was good. My coworkers either buy lunch out, or we have a cafeteria at work which doesn't have great variety. Frankly, the cafeteria food doesn't taste good. Anyway, I had an apple and an orange packed, so I ate the orange with my lunch and then I kept my apple and ate it later in the afternoon. That was very nice too. It kept me from going to the vending machine and getting a candy bar when I was hungry."

**Coach Carl:** "Then you really went above and beyond with this goal. So it was a treat to have a lunch that you knew you were going to enjoy?"

**Wendy Well:** "Yes and because it was there and it was easy—normally, if you put an apple and a candy bar on my desk, I would go for the candy bar, but I think because I had eaten a good healthy lunch and then because the fruit was there, it was just easier I guess."

**Coach Carl:** "And, what happened on Wednesday and Friday when you weren't able to take the lunch?"

**Wendy Well:** "On Tuesday, I had just gotten back from a business trip and was really tired and got to bed late. So when I got up on Wednesday I actually did think about it. And by Friday, I had kind of gotten out of the habit of it again and I just thought that everything I bought last weekend was getting old so I didn't pack it."

**Coach Carl:** "I hear you beating yourself up a little bit for that, and perhaps we can come back to that at some point in the conversation after we've finished checking in on the goals. I'm also hearing that it just wasn't as convenient for you on Wednesday and Friday."

## COACHING CASE Continued

**Wendy Well:** "Right."

**Coach Carl:** "Some things weren't in place for that to happen. So what do you know now about yourself or the goal that you didn't know last week when you set this goal?"

**Wendy Well:** "I guess what I know is that I need the time, I need the pre-planning, and I need to have it organized if I want to make it work. I also know that when I get tired, I don't make good choices. I don't put the energy into doing things ahead of time. That's going to happen sometimes."

**Coach Carl:** "And there are other times that you do put the energy into it, and you plan, and that's met with great success. So tell me about your percentage of success here."

**Wendy Well:** "I guess that would be about 33%."

This allows the client to be flexible and adaptable, perhaps modifying his or her three-month goals and/or resetting the start or end date if the goals are too challenging, if a major disruption has emerged, or if a bigger challenge is necessary.

This is an opportunity for the coach to ask a client to zoom out and confirm that his or her vision is still connected to the three-month goals and take stock of what the client has learned along the journey thus far (Table 11.4).

| Table 11.4 | Three-Month Goal Review |
|---|---|
| Validates the relevance of the client's vision and connection to three-month goals |
| Asks about the client's best learning or growth experience with his or her three-month goals |
| Asks about the client's level of engagement commitment with his or her goals and whether he or she wants to revise them |
| Affirms the client's strengths, abilities, or growth |

## COACHING CASE

**Three-Month Goal Review**

**Coach Carl:** "In what ways do these three-month goals support you in getting to that powerful vision that you set a few months ago?"

**Wendy Well:** "I know these three-months goals are the direct pathway to having more energy, getting more accomplished, and feeling better in general."

**Coach Carl:** "Great. And, are these the goals you want to continue working toward?"

**Wendy Well:** "Yes I do."

**Coach Carl:** "And as you've worked toward these for the last several weeks, what have you learned about yourself in the process?"

**Wendy Well:** "I've learned that I can make changes. It's not an all-or-nothing type of thing. But I've also learned that it's easy to get sidetracked and postpone important things."

**Coach Carl:** "It sounds like you've learned about the importance of having a plan in place and some priorities in place."

**Wendy Well:** "Oh yes! You have helped me unpack and be mindful of the nitty-gritty details of starting new habits."

**Coach Carl:** "That's my job! I've seen you make such tremendous progress in the last several weeks. It's been exciting to be a part of that process. I really admire your tenacity through this. I'm excited to see you continue to take the next steps for those three-month goals. Well done!"

# Generate New Learning with the Generative Moment

After the goal progress has been reviewed, the area that clients are most stimulated by or struggling with typically becomes evident. Sometimes, it is success and excitement that carries them forward into a generative moment (see Chapter 10). Other times, it is a challenge, ambivalence, anxiety, or uncertainty. Either way, coaches will want to spend extra time with clients around these areas (Table 11.5). These are the big rocks around which clients want to move in generative moments.

## Goal Setting

Goal setting (or the design of experiments) emerges naturally on the tail of a generative moment. When clients have elevated their self-efficacy or belief in their ability to accomplish a task or goal, especially in an area that is important to them, they want to set new goals for the week ahead that will keep them moving forward. It is important to be sure the goals are measurable, owned by the client, and reinforced by as many support structures as possible (Table 11.6).

| Table 11.6 | Goal Setting |
| --- | --- |
| Asks the client to choose a goal that is important and that he or she is ready to pursue |
| Explores the support, structure, or environments needed to ensure success and handle challenges |
| Assists the client to refine goal to be a SMART behavioral goal |
| Uses confidence ruler to improve the client's confidence in reaching that goal |
| Asks client to restate goals |
| Affirms client's ability to achieve his or her goals |

In addition to the goals that flow out of the generative moment collaboration, it is important to help clients set goals in all areas of interest or concern.

A written summary of goals is ideally exchanged between coaches and clients after every coaching session. This serves to facilitate the accountability process and to keep the forward momentum from week to week. Initially, it may be helpful for the coach to write up the plan—vision, three-month goals, and first week's goals—in order to demonstrate how to summarize a succinct and compelling plan.

## Session Close

As with the session close for initial sessions, it is important to end on a positive note, expressing appreciation for the client's work and capturing what the client learned. The coach can also take the opportunity to ask for feedback on how to make the coaching session even more effective in promoting the client's forward progress (Figure 11.1) before scheduling the next session (Table 11.7).

## Handling Client Challenges

Although every client and every coaching interaction is unique, there are some common challenges that can happen in the coaching process. It is valuable to be aware of some of the common situations

| Table 11.5 | Generative Moment |
| --- | --- |
| Collaborates with the client to identify the topic on which to work on, where he or she has aroused emotional energy and interest |
| Asks for permission to explore and work on the topic now |
| Encourages the client to describe what he or she really wants now in relation to the topic |
| Explores the strengths or values the client can leverage to move forward |
| Explores the environments the client can leverage to move forward |
| Explores decisional balance and develops discrepancy when the client demonstrates ambivalence |
| Engages the client in creative brainstorming of pathways forward |
| Expresses confidence in the client's ability to move forward |

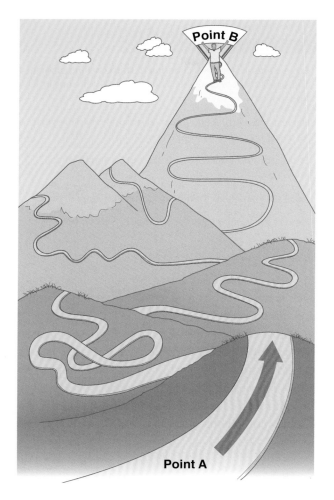

**Figure 11.1.** Celebrating success and championing the client.

| Table 11.7 | Session Close |
| --- | --- |
| Communicates an appreciation of the client's work in the session | |
| Discovers and reflects what the client learned in the session | |
| Asks for feedback on how future coaching sessions would best support client's path | |
| Schedules next session | |

*Situation:* Clients are starting to get bored.
*Approach:* Add variety to generative moment discussions, offer a new assessment, and explore other domains for change and goals.

*Situation:* Clients are not making their change process a priority (may be manifested in excuses as well as missed and/or late appointments).
*Approach:* Share your observations, express empathy, and inquire as to what could make their visions and goals more of a priority. Share with clients the value of taking small, incremental steps (e.g., how short bursts of exercise are beneficial).

*Situation:* Clients realize that coaches are not magicians, and they become disillusioned as to how much work it will take to make changes.
*Approach:* Normalize their experiences (everyone goes through this). Emphasize smaller steps. Share your confidence in the process with clients, and assist clients with creating action plans that they find engaging and can be successful with in meeting weekly goals.

*Situation:* Clients are not attempting the behaviors they set for themselves as SMART goals on a weekly basis.
*Approach:* Look for what is working in client behaviors in order to set new goals that clients will experience as a fresh start. Probe deeply for inspiring motivators. If situation persists, discuss the matter with a mentor coach to determine next steps.

*Situation:* Client is not at the 50% point of their three-month goals at week 6.
*Approach:* Reassess three-month goals with your client to make sure they are realistic. Revisit the

clients might experience along the way and possible approaches that can be taken.

*Situation:* Clients may tend toward being over-zealous and unrealistic.
*Approach:* Carefully monitor goals to help clients keep them realistic.

*Situation:* Clients are slow to become motivated and do not make noticeable progress.
*Approach:* Address readiness to change or motivational problems through AI and motivational interviewing (MI). Discover strengths, build self-efficacy, weigh the pros and cons of change, modify environmental conditions, try new strategies to overcome roadblocks, and reconfirm or find new motivators.

vision to reignite its power. Discuss situation with a mentor coach for new ideas for generating success.

*Situation:* Clients get discouraged by not seeing results in several areas.

*Approach:* First, focus on what is working and on the client's strengths. Then, spend extra time discussing the areas in which expectations have not been met, and create a plan for improvement. Try different tools and resources. Discuss options with a mentor coach.

| Table 11.8 | Coaching Program Close |
|---|---|
| Explore reasons for client choosing to stop coaching program and/or ask client to complete a brief survey like the one in Appendix B. |
| Harvest and celebrate his or her learning, and explore what he or she may want to consider next. |
| Encourage client to keep making progress and to let you know how he or she is doing. |
| Ask if you may check in with him or her from time to time. |
| Express your gratitude for the privilege to work with the client. |

## Coaching Program Refresh or Close

The three-month point in coaching is a good time to review and renew the coaching program. It is a time to celebrate the achievement of milestones, consider developing a new three-month plan, modify coaching session frequency, and/or renew your client's commitment to the coaching program.

When a coaching program comes to a close, it's time to harvest and celebrate a client's accomplishments and learning. A coaching session can be dedicated to deeper reflection, unpacking the full experience to learn from it. What went well? What sustainable mindset and behavior changes were made? What impact are the changes having on a client's life? What's next? How can the coach support a client in his or her next phase?

Perhaps the client wants to consolidate what he or she has learned and end the coaching partnership for now. Perhaps the client wants to continue the coaching program with a new focus. Either way, it's a good moment to have the client complete a coaching program evaluation survey along the lines summarized in Appendix B. It may also be helpful to track post-coaching outcomes one or more years later to confirm the coaching impact and track record (Table 11.8).

Coaches and clients often continue a connection for many years. A coach can send a birthday message or check in periodically on a client's well-being. They may meet once in a while. A happy client is an excellent source of referrals and may even wish to restart a coaching program on a new domain at a later date.

Most of all, a coach can take time to reflect on what went well and consider what areas of coaching skills, processes, and impacts present opportunities for professional growth and development. The journey of learning and growth never ends for coaches and clients alike.

## References

Berna, J. (2013). Wellness coaching outcomes in a case report of a Native American diabetic male. *Global Advances in Health and Medicine, 2*(4), 62–67.

Brown, T. (2008). Design thinking. *Harvard Business Review, 86*(6), 84–92, 141.

Fredrickson, B. L. (2009). *Positivity: Groundbreaking research reveals how to embrace the hidden strength of positive emotions, overcome, negativity, and thrive.* New York: Crown.

Galantino, M., Schmid, P., Milos, A., Leonard, S., Botis, S., Dagan, C., . . . Mao, J. (2009). Longitudinal benefits of wellness coaching interventions for cancer survivors. *International Journal of Interdisciplinary Social Sciences, 4*(10), 41–58.

McGloin, H., Timmons, F., Coates, V., & Boore, J. (2014). A case study approach to the examination of a telephone-based health coaching intervention in facilitating behaviour change for adults with type 2 diabetes. *Journal of Clinical Nursing.* Advance online publication. http://dx.doi.org/10.1111/jocn.12692.

Polak, R., Dill, D., Abrahamson, M., Pojednic, R., & Phillips, E. (2014). Improving consumption of healthy food in a patient with diabetes through wellness coaching. *Global Advances in Health and Medicine, 3*(6), 42–48.

Roy, B., Lisowski, C., & Roberts, P. (2014). Wellness coaching with physician-referred patients with chronic health conditions. *Journal of Clinical Exercise Physiology, 3*(1), 9–15.

Schwartz, J. (2013). Wellness coaching for obesity. *Global Advances in Health and Medicine, 2*(4), 1–3.

Sforzo, G. (2013). Wellness coaching for Ithaca College employees. *Global Advances in Health and Medicine, 2*(3), 58–64.

Sforzo, G., Kaye, M., Ayers, G., Talbert, M., & Hill, M. (2014). Effective 4.1 tobacco cessation via health coaching: An institutional case report. *Global Advances in Health and Medicine, 3*(5), 37–44.

Sherman, R., Crocker, B., Dill, D., & Judge, D. (2013). Health coaching integration into primary care for the treatment of obesity. *Global Advances in Health and Medicine, 2*(4), 1–3.

# Appendix A:
# Coaching Program Guidelines

## Phase 1: Prospect Stage

E-mail personal welcome and introduction and articles as appropriate.

Discuss what is coaching and what is not.

Introduce coach's biography.

Discuss program protocol, fees, and payment terms.

## Phase 2: Program Startup

### Set Expectations

Share, discuss, and agree coaching agreement principles or template.

Confirm confidentiality and record keeping.

Clarify expectations regarding logistics (e.g., payments, scheduling, rescheduling, and length of sessions).

Share assessment for client to complete.

### Prepare for Session

Prepare: Review client assessment results and client communication.

Get present: Practice mindfulness, set intention, and connect to purpose.

Get curious: Consider initial strengths-based inquiries.

### Session Opening

Welcome and thank you

Thank client for completing assessment.

Review the session agenda: Confirm client's expectations and priorities, review an assessment, gather additional information, create vision, and design goals.

### Explore Assessment

Find positive aspects to emphasize and share from the client's assessments.

Ask client what he or she learned about him or herself by completing the assessments.

Ask client what questions he or she has after completing the assessments.

Gather missing information.

Discuss client's medical history and need for physician release if applicable.

### Design a Vision

Explain the value of creating a vision.

Ask what is most important to the client right now and what makes him or her thrive.

Collaborate to identify the client strengths: Review success stories, discuss what is working now, and discover what gives the client pride.

Discover the client's motivators: Ask about the benefits of making changes now, and ask about the driving force behind the desire to change now.

Ask about the client's vision (hopes, wishes, and dreams) for health, fitness, or wellness.

Support the client in visualizing his or her vision and describing it in detail.

Use confidence ruler to assess and improve self-efficacy.

Ask what challenges would be met and what things would be possible if the vision were a reality.

Discover previous positive experiences with elements of the vision.

Identify the strengths and values that could be used to reach the vision.

Explore the support (people, resources, systems, and environments) needed to ensure success and handle challenges.

Ask the client to state and commit to the vision.

### Design Three-Month Goals

Explain the nature and value of setting three-month goals.

Brainstorm consistent behaviors that would lead to the achievement of the vision.

Ask the client to choose several behavioral goals that are most important to pursue.

Confirm the connection of the behaviors to the vision.

Assist the client in developing SMART behavioral goals and an experimental learning mindset.

### Design Action Plan

Ask the client to choose goals/experiments that are important next steps toward three-month behavioral goals.

Assist the client in designing SMART behavioral goals.

Use confidence ruler to improve the client's confidence in reaching the goal.

Explore the client's strengths and support (people, resources, systems, and environments) needed to ensure success and handle challenges.

Ask the client to restate and commit to SMART goals.

Affirm the client's ability to achieve the goals and emphasize learning/growth mindset.

### Session Close

Express appreciation for the client's work.

Discover and reflect what the client learned.

Confirm that the client is ready, confident, and committed to take agreed on actions.

Ask for feedback on how future coaching sessions would best support the client's path.

Clarify expectations regarding payments, scheduling, rescheduling, and length of sessions.

Schedule the next session.

### Phase 3: Ongoing Coaching Program

### Prepare for Session

Prepare: Review notes from previous session(s).

Get present: Practice mindfulness, set intention, and connect to purpose.

Get curious: Consider initial strengths-based inquiries.

### Session Opening

Ask how the client is right now in this moment.

Use reflections to show appreciation and understanding of client's state.

Ask the client to share the best thing that happened from previous week(s).

Reflect something positive about the client (e.g., highlights, strengths, or emotions).

Ask client to select the first weekly goal to be discussed.

### Actions/Experimental Goal Review

Explore full experience with weekly goal starting with the positive.

Use reflections to show listening and understanding of the goal experience.

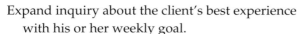

Expand inquiry about the client's best experience with his or her weekly goal.

Respond to client challenges with judgment-free reflections and inquiries.

Ask what the client learned from his or her experience.

Affirm the client's strengths, values, choices, and/or situations.

Inquire about the client's percentage of success.

### Three-Month Goal Check-In

Validate the relevance of the client's vision and connection to three-month goals.

Ask about the client's best learning or growth experience with his or her three-month goals.

Ask about the client's level of engagement and commitment with his or her goals.

Affirm the client's strengths, abilities, or growth.

### Generative Moment

Collaborate with the client to identify the topic on which to work on, where he or she has aroused emotional energy and interest.

Ask for permission to explore and work on the topic now.

Encourage the client to describe what he or she really wants now, in relation to the topic.

Explore the strengths or values the client can leverage to move forward.

Explore the environments the client can leverage to move forward.

Explore decisional balance and develop discrepancy when the client demonstrates ambivalence.

Engage the client in creative brainstorming of pathways forward.

Express confidence in the client's ability to move forward.

### Goal Setting

Ask the client to choose a goal that is important.

Assist the client in designing a SMART behavioral goal/experiment.

Use a confidence ruler to improve the client's confidence in reaching the goal.

Explore the support (people, resources, systems, and environments) needed to ensure success and handle challenges.

Ask the client to restate and commit to the SMART goal.

Affirm the client's ability to achieve the goal.

### Session Close

Communicate an appreciation of the client's work in the session.

Discover and reflect what the client learned in the session.

Ask for feedback on how future coaching sessions would best support client's path.

Schedule next session.

## Phase 4: Coaching Program Close

Explore reasons for the client choosing to stop coaching program and/or ask the client to complete a brief survey like the one in Appendix B.

Harvest and celebrate his or her learning, and explore what they may want to consider next.

Encourage client to keep making progress and to let you know how they are doing.

Ask if you may check in with the client from time to time.

Express your gratitude for the privilege to work with the client.

## Appendix B:

# Coaching Program Feedback Survey

Coach's Name:

Client's Name:

Coaching Start Date:

Please rate your coach's competence on a scale of 1–10: 10 = Very Competent; 1 = Very Incompetent. Please feel free to add any comments.

|  | Rating | Comments |
|---|---|---|
| Knowledge: | | |
| Helpfulness: | | |
| Empathy and connection: | | |
| Quality of change support: | | |
| Quality of guidance: | | |
| Quality of resources: | | |

Effectiveness:

Other comments:

Areas for improvement:

In what ways has coaching benefited or changed you the most? Describe "before" and "after" if possible.

What goal is most important to you now?

*Please comment on how coaching has benefited you in any of the following areas:*

Confidence:

Motivation:

Energy:

Work performance/productivity:

Exercise habits:

Eating habits:

Sleep:

Stress management:

Self-compassion:

Health:

Life satisfaction:

What are your coach's best qualities?

How could your coach improve?

How does your coaching experience differ from your expectations?

# CHAPTER 12

# The Thriving Coach

*"Don't ask what the world needs. Ask what makes you come alive, and go do it. Because what the world needs is people who have come alive."*

—HOWARD THURMAN

## Last Words from Coach Meg

It's all well and good for coaches to help their clients grow, change, and thrive. However, a coach's integrity depends on walking the walk, continually growing and learning, and, even better, to model thriving. As we have explored throughout this manual, there are many models and constructs for human thriving and well-being. Let's do a quick tour and consider how coaches can use this manual's lessons in order to thrive themselves. Then we will leave you with a provocative new model and a call to action.

In Chapter 1, we introduced self-determination theory (Deci & Ryan, 2002), which is a model for human thriving. A coach thrives if his or her needs for autonomy, relatedness, and competence are met. In Chapter 2, we explored key coaching skills that underpin the evocative collaboration of coaching, which supports the thriving of both coach and client in the moment. Not only are clients energized and inspired by a generative coaching session, coaches are too. These are often the peak moments in a coach's work life. Chapter 3 helps coaches consider new ways to fully engage and manifest their strengths in coaching and beyond. New tools for navigating and settling negative emotions are

explored in Chapter 4, and these are just as helpful for coaches as for clients—learning to suffer well and quickly finding the calm in an emotional storm. In Chapter 5, we introduced the field of positive psychology, dedicated to studying what makes humans thrive, mostly mentally. The field's founder, Martin Seligman (2011), made a call to action for 51% of the population to flourish by 2051, an increase from around 20% of the population today, through positive emotions, engagement, better relationships, and purpose beyond self. Coaches are leading the way and inspiring their clients to do the same.

Digging out autonomous heartfelt motivation and life force and pouring that motivational energy into getting better, improving competence and confidence, explored in Chapter 6, is a recipe for thriving while changing and growing every day. Coaches can do this by trying out new coaching tools or taking risks in coaching sessions. Chapter 7 explores the characteristics of early stages of readiness to change when people may feel stuck in chronic contemplation. Coaches can recognize their personal readiness quickly and stay focused on new habits of mind and body that they are ready, willing, and able to develop. They can set more intimidating goals aside. There is no shortage of assessments of various aspects and constructs of well-being, a few of which we introduced in Chapter 8 to help coaches continually take stock and explore new opportunities to upgrade their own well-being.

Coaches benefit from designing visions, goals, and experiments as much as clients do. They can model focused attention on a thoughtful future-oriented, flexible, and buttoned-down approach to personal change, as we explore in Chapter 9. In Chapters 10 and 11, in which we describe the processes of coaching during sessions, we show how clients design visions, goals, and fully unpack their experience toward their goals. A key takeaway for coaches is to work with a coach themselves on a regular basis in order to experience the creative generativity, shifts, and transformations in mindset that happen consistently with a skilled coach.

Before we say goodbye, which is never easy even when writing a book, we want to share a provocative new approach to thriving, and also to emotional intelligence, mindfulness, and coaching, explored in a published hypothesis paper: *Coaching the Multiplicity of Mind: A Strengths-Based Approach* (Moore, 2013), the basis for a book underway, which follows our first book *Organize Your Mind, Organize Your Life* (Hammerness & Moore, 2011). No doubt this second edition of the *Coaching Psychology Manual* will be out of date in several years, and new constructs and research-based coaching tools will be added to the next edition. In the meantime, this model offers a new lens and contributes to a larger dialogue on what it means to thrive.

# Human Thriving—Nine Primary Capacities

The basis of the model is that the psyche is made up of a set of discrete human needs, drives, or capacities that manifest as sub-personalities, all together creating an ongoing inner dialogue and ever-changing kaleidoscope of agendas and concerns. These capacities communicate their agendas via voices, emotions, and physical sensations, continuously signaling whether needs are being met or not. Thriving from this perspective happens when we are able to decode our genetically based needs and capacities, meet those needs, and use the capacities as fully as possible. With that in mind, we describe nine primary capacities that together contribute to human thriving. These capacities won't seem new or surprising, as we have touched on the themes throughout this manual. It's a testament to the coaching field that coaches have integrated the major evidence-based themes of human thriving into the coaching toolbox. The summary that follows is adapted from an International Coach Federation *Coaching World* article titled "From Surviving to Thriving" (Moore, 2014).

## Body Regulation

Along with all living organisms, humans have a primary need for a healthy and calm equilibrium of our physiological systems—a need to move from chaos to homeostasis over and over. As Stephen W. Porges (2007) outlines in his polyvagal theory, our bodies seek a balance of exertion with rest and recharge. They strive for homeostasis, stability, safety, health, and a robust autonomic nervous system, balancing sympathetic (stress) and parasympathetic (rest and recover) activity. Listening to the body's signals tells us when it's time to calm the nervous system, which calms the mind and improves brain function in the short term and delays disease and early death in the long term. Given the epidemics of lifestyle-related chronic disease, the body regulator is a voice that is getting drowned out by other needs described in the following text. Coaches can help clients tune into their "body intelligence," learning to listen to basic needs for balance, and physical energy and health (Gavin & Moore, 2010) by encouraging them to pay attention to the signals of the body within coaching sessions through mindfulness and other practices of intention.

An existential question posed by this part of our psyches is "Do I have the physical and other resources I need to live fully?"

## Autonomy

Psychologists Edward L. Deci and Richard M. Ryan (2002), who have studied human motivation for three decades, leading to their robust theory of self-determination, conclude that autonomy—the drive to march to one's own drummer—is the first, primary organismic need. To thrive, we need to be authentic and author a life aligned with our values. Autonomous motivation that taps into one's life force is not only a stand-alone force for thriving; it is the type of motivation that enables elusive habits, including healthy eating, exercise, and weight loss and maintenance, to be sustained. It is a far superior fuel source to external motivators, such as incentives, prizes, or the fear-based "stick" of external or internal critics. An existential question posed by this part of our psyches is "Am I doing the right things in my life, marching to my own drummer, aligned with my heartfelt values?"

## Making Meaning and Purpose

Clinical psychologist Paul Wong (2014) is one of the most passionate spokespeople for the importance of making meaning and purpose beyond oneself in each moment, in each domain of life, and over the arc of a lifetime. In his chapter, "Viktor Frankl's Meaning Seeking Model and Positive Psychology," Wong keeps alive the legendary psychiatrist and Holocaust survivor's story, as told in *Man's Search for Meaning* (Frankl, 2006). The story told is how an unshakable purpose was essential to surviving four Nazi concentration camps. A sense of a higher purpose is a potent source of life fuel, especially when times are tough. For example, a team of researchers at Chicago's Rush Alzheimer's Disease Center and Rush University Medical Center found that a sense of life purpose significantly improves cognitive function in people with Alzheimer's disease. Meanwhile, Barbara Fredrickson and colleagues made scientific headlines in 2013 with an experiment, now repeated twice, which showed that people with a low level of life purpose had three impaired gene pathways in their immune systems, whereas people with a high level of life purpose had healthy gene expression of these three gene pathways. Our genes may reward us for being connected to a cause larger than ourselves by fighting off cold and flu viruses and other invaders that could make us ill. An existential question posed by this part of our psyches

is "Am I contributing to making the world a better place in small or larger ways?"

## Relationships

Serving others, taking care of others, being compassionate and kind, and at times choosing to put the needs of others ahead of our own are important sources of human thriving. Indeed, Deci and Flaste (1996) identify relatedness as another innate psychological need. In *Love 2.0: How Our Supreme Emotion Affects Everything We Feel, Think, Do, and Become,* Fredrickson (2013) encourages us to "make love all day long"; in other words, to infuse each moment in another's company with your full attention, your head and heart in it together. In addition to simply feeling good, sharing positive emotions with others creates micro-moments of connection, which calm the nervous system and improve brain function. Over time, these micro-moments accumulate to help delay disease and avoid early death. Compassion for negative emotions experienced by ourselves and others is a soothing balm. Just like crying babies, negative emotions need a warm, appreciative embrace to settle and allow us to get on with our day. An existential question posed by this part of our psyches is "Am I helping others meet their needs, channel their drives, honor their values, and use their capacities, also for concerns beyond self-interest?"

## Confidence and Competence

Confidence—what Albert Bandura (1997) put on the map as the psychological term "self-efficacy"—is a strong predictor of successful performance in work goals and creating new health habits. As Henry Ford stated, "Whether you think you can, or you think you can't—you're right." Deci and Ryan's (2002) self-determination theory identifies competence as one of three primary organismic needs, suggesting that acquiring new knowledge and skills, applying our chief strengths, and continually growing confidence are all vital lifetime pursuits. A well-being-focused coaching engagement or self-coaching process can get us on the right track, instilling confidence in the ability to combine a full work and family life with a focus on self-care and well-being; this includes exercising safely, cooking well, keeping a healthy and stable weight, sleeping peacefully, and taming the overwhelming frenzy brought on by a life switch stuck in the "on" position. An existential question posed by this part of our psyches is "Am I getting better, more competent, and confident?"

## Curiosity and New Experience Seeking

Psychologist Todd Kashdan (2012) asserts that curiosity is a primary driver of human well-being, writing, "When we experience curiosity, we are willing to leave the familiar and routine and take risks, even if it makes us feel anxious and uncomfortable. Curious explorers are comfortable with the risks of taking on new challenges. Instead of trying desperately to explain and control our world, as a curious explorer, we embrace uncertainty and see our lives as an enjoyable quest to discover, learn, and grow."

The primary need for new experiences to explore, learn, and change is easy to see in curious children but is often squashed by the demands of adult life. This is an important capacity for adapting to an ever-changing world: being ever-curious and never taking anything for granted, including one's assumptions and beliefs. In fact, Kashdan notes that declining curiosity is one of the important early signs of dementia and Alzheimer's disease. Coaches support clients in shifting to the perspective that life is just one big set of experiments with unpredictable outcomes. An existential question posed by this part of our psyches is "Am I open and curious and engaged in life's adventures?"

## Creativity

We also quickly see in children a primary capacity to be creative, generative, imaginative, and spontaneous, but these traits often seem out of reach for adults, dealing with overscheduled days and overstretched minds. Creativity improves both mental and physical health. It often works best when our brains are unleashed to wander about, unplugged from deadlines and goals. This part of us has fun brainstorming, playing games, and being impulsive. When in full flight, it produces flow states that

Mihaly Csikszentmihalyi (2008) describes as key to optimal well-being—those moments in which we are enjoying an activity so much that we lose track of time. Without undue effort, we execute the activity to the best of our abilities. While the workplace is the best place for experiencing regular flow states, most people do not let themselves enjoy flow states every day because their minds are constrained by overwhelming to-do lists and distractions. An existential question posed by this part of our psyches is "Am I generative, coming up with new ideas and possibilities to address life's challenges?"

## Executive Function

Thank goodness humans have a primary capacity to be organized, to plan, to regulate emotions and impulses, and stay on track to get through to-do lists and meet goals. This capacity is highly polished in the workplace (although often at the expense of other capacities previously described). Those with attention deficits need to work harder to build self-regulation skills and to learn to set aside disruptive emotions, impulses, and distractions so that they get the important things done. Executive function gets a powerful boost when people tame their emotional frenzy, exercise regularly, sleep well, and eat a healthy diet. An existential question posed by this part of our psyches is "Am I doing things right or well?"

## Standard Setting

As the most social animals on the planet, humans share a primary need for approval, appreciation, validation, and fair treatment by others. No man is an island. We want to be accepted and valued by our family, friends, colleagues, and communities. This capacity allows us to set the bar or standard, to set goals for our performance, and then to evaluate and judge that performance in ourselves and others across all domains of life, from getting good grades at school to dying well. "Am I good enough?" it asks.

At its worst, this capacity is difficult to please. It can be an inner critic, scanning for flaws and faults, or a perfectionist, ever raising the bar. Sadly, a recent study reported that only 11% of women over the age of 50 report satisfaction with their bodies

(Runfola et al., 2013), their inner critics depleting their self-esteem every time they look in a mirror. At its best, the inner standard setter is accepting and content, setting the bar to challenge performance while adopting a learning mindset when performance falls short. This state of contentment is difficult for many to find in an achievement-oriented culture and 24/7 pace. An existential question posed by this part of our psyches in addition to "Am I good enough" is "Am I doing enough?"

When humans welcome, appreciate, and honor all of these discrete and often conflicting needs and agendas, the inner ambivalence and conflicts can settle, even if just a little, bringing more thriving and equanimity. Coaches can help people accept and advocate for all parts of themselves, discover underused capacities, and strive to meet more of their needs more of the time.

## The Call for Coaches

In closing, the field of health and wellness coaches, and all health professionals who are applying coaching skills, face an enormous task ahead—that of improving the thriving, mental and physical, of the human race. Roughly 20% of adults are thriving today, so there is a long way to go (Kobau, Sniezek, Zack, Lucas, & Burns, 2010). Unleashing human thriving is the life calling, the higher purpose, for a whole new generation of the thousands of health and wellness coaches we aim to teach and inspire throughout this manual. A small army of health and wellness coaches has emerged in the past decade to focus on unleashing positive mental and physical well-being and making a dent in the epidemics of chronic disease and obesity. We need all hands on deck—not only coaches but anyone who wants to join this effort. Let's thrive first, and then help everyone we touch get there, too.

Onward and upward.

## References

Bandura, A. (1997). *Self-efficacy: The exercise of control.* New York: W. H. Freeman.

Csikszentmihalyi, M. (2008). *Flow: The psychology of optimal experience.* New York: Harper Perennial Modern Classics.

Deci, E., & Flaste, R. (1996). *Why we do what we do: Understanding self-motivation.* New York: Penguin.

Deci, E. L., & Ryan, R. M. (2002). *Handbook of self-determination research.* New York: University of Rochester Press.

Frankl, V. (2006). *Man's search for meaning.* Boston, MA: Beacon Press.

Fredrickson, B. (2013). *Love 2.0: How our supreme emotion affects everything we feel, think, do and become.* New York: Hudson Press.

Fredrickson, B., Grewen, K., Coffey, K., Algoe, S., Firestine, A., Arevalo, J., . . . Cole, S. (2013). A functional genomic perspective on human well-being. *Proceedings of the National Academy of Sciences of the United States of America, 110,* 13684–13689.

Gavin, J., & Moore, M. (2010). *Body intelligence: A guide to self-attunement.* Retrieved April 27, 2015 from http://www.ideafit.com/fitness-library/body-intelligence-a-guide-to

Hammerness, P., & Moore, M. (2011). *Organize your mind, organize your life: Train your brain to get more done in less time.* New York: Harlequin.

Kashdan, T. (2009). *Curious?: Discover the missing ingredient to a fulfilling life.* New York: HarperCollins.

Kobau, R., Sniezek, J., Zack, M., Lucas, R., & Burns, A. (2010). Well-being assessment: An evaluation of well-being scales for public health and population estimates of well-being among US adults. *Applied Psychology: Health and Well-Being, 2,* 272–297.

Moore, M. (2013). Coaching the multiplicity of mind: A strengths-based model. *Global Advances in Health and Medicine, 2*(4), 78–84.

Moore, M. (2014). From surviving to thriving [Web log post]. Retrieved April 27, 2015 from http://coach federation.org/blog/index.php/2090/

Porges, S. (2007). The polyvagal perspective. *Biological Psychology, 74*(2), 116–143.

Runfola, C. D., Von Holle, A., Peat, C. M., Gagne, D. A., Brownley, K. A., Hofmeier, S. M., & Bulik, C. M. (2013). Characteristics of women with body size satisfaction at midlife: Results of the Gender and Body Image (GABI) Study. *Journal of Women and Aging, 25*(4), 287–304.

Seligman, M. (2011). *Flourish: A visionary new understanding of happiness and well-being.* New York: Free Press.

Wong, P. T. P. (2014). Viktor Frankl's meaning seeking model and positive psychology. In A. Batthyany & P. Russo-Netzer (Eds.), *Meaning in existential and positive psychology.* New York: Springer Publishing.

# Index

Note: Page numbers followed by *f* and *t* indicate figures and tables, respectively.

## A

Abrahamson, M., 155
Academy of Nutrition and Dietetics, 120
Accountability, 158–159
ACSM. *See* American College of Sports Medicine
*ACSM's Guidelines for Exercise Testing and Prescription*, 120
*Action Coaching* (Dotlich and Cairo), 28
Action level, of Mount Lasting Change Model
  behavioral steps, 109
  problem solving, 109
  rewards, 109
Action stage, of change, 98–99
Affective listening, 34
Affective states, 88
Affirmation
  as being skill, 46–47
  unfailing, 145
AI. *See* Appreciative inquiry
Alzheimer disease, 86, 175, 176
Ambivalence, 109–110
American College of Sports Medicine (ACSM), 120
American Psychological Association (APA), 63
Amplified reflections, 84
Amygdala, 56
Anorexia, 120
Anticipatory principle, 66–67
Anxiety disorders, 120
APA. *See* American Psychological Association
Appreciative inquiry (AI), 77, 82, 127, 133–134
  coaching relationship and, 74–75
  5-D cycle of, 67–71, 67*f*
  five principles of, 65–67, 65*f*
    anticipatory principle, 66–67
    constructionist principle, 66
    poetic principle, 67
    positive principle, 66
    simultaneity principle, 66
  generative moments and, 147, 148
  value of, 71–72
  verbal persuasion and, 89
  well-being assessments and, 121–122
*The Art of Possibility* (Zander, R. and Zander, B.), 48
Assessments
  for coaching, 115–118

  HRAs, 114
  Quickie Well-Being Assessment, 116, 117*f*
  readiness to change, 104, 105*t*, 152
  value of, 113–115
    autonomy and, 115
    caution in use of, 114–115
  of well-being, 118–124
Athletic development, 21
Attractive indicators, for generative moments, 142
Australian Psychological Society, 11
Authenticity
  as being skill, 48–49
  trust and rapport and, 32
Autonomous motivation, 14, 78–80, 175
Autonomy, 5, 12, 139
  assessments and, 115
  human thriving and, 174–175
Aversive indicators, 142
Awareness
  creating, 114
  MAAS, 116
  open, 45
  self-awareness, 107
Ayers, G., 155

## B

Bach, Richard, 63
Bandura, Albert, 12, 87, 89, 175
Beauty, appreciation of, 52–53
Behavioral factors, in SCT, 87
Behavioral goals, 132–135
  change and, 103
  examples of, 136*t*
  first experiment or goal, 135*t*
  low, 135
  measurable, 133
  performance, 16
  realistic, 133
  reasons for setting, 133–134
  review of, 159*t*
    accountability and, 158–159
    three-month check-in and, 159–161, 161*t*
  setting, 162
  SMART, 16, 71, 133
Behavioral steps, 109
Behavior change
  client support and, 102–104
    operant conditioning and, 103–104
    self-efficacy and, 103

  coaching skills for, 101*t*, 102*t*
  decisional balance and, 82–83
  general suggestions for, 109–111
  Mount Lasting Change Model, 93, 106–109, 107*f*, 114
  processes of, 15–16, 100–102
  readiness to change, 118–119
    assessment, 104, 105*t*, 152
  self-change, 94
  stages of, 100*f*
    action, 98–99
    contemplation, 96–97
    maintenance, 99–100
    precontemplation, 94–96
    preparation, 97–98
  TTM and, 15, 90, 93–94, 100, 118, 134
*Being Genuine: Stop Being Nice, Start Being Real* (d'Ansembourg), 49
Being skills, 44*f*
  affirmation, 46–47
  authenticity, 48–49
  calm, 47
  courage, 48–49
  empathy, 45–46
  mindfulness, 44–45, 45*f*
  playfulness, 48
  warmth, 46
  zest, 47–48
Bennis, Warren, 67
Berna, J., 156
Best experience, 68–69
Best self, 106, 109
Board Certified Coach credential, 22
Body
  generative moments and, 146
  regulation of, 174
Body intelligence, 45, 174
Bombeck, Erma, 113
Boore, J., 155
Botelho, Richard, 83
Boundaries
  couching principles and, 128
  values and, 108
Boyle, P. A., 86
Brain
  Alzheimer disease and, 86
  amygdala, 56
  growth-promoting relationships and, 13–14
  mindfulness and, 45*f*
  perceptive reflections and, 37

Brainsets, 13, 45
  envision, 16
Brainstorming, 135–137
  generative moments and, 144–145,
    149–151
Bravery, 51
Briggs, Dorothy Corkville, 93
British Psychological Society, 11
Brown, Brené, 57
Brown, K., 116
Brown, T., 126
Brue, Susan, 116
Buck, Dave, 27, 39, 47, 89
"Building a Practically Useful Theory of
  Goal Setting and Task Motivation: A 35-
  Year Odyssey" (Locke and Latham), 133
Bungee jumping, 89
Burnout, 19
Business coaches, 1

**C**
Cairo, Peter, 28
Calm, 47
Cancer, 3, 7
Carson, Shelley, 13, 16, 45
Case Western Reserve University, 65
CDC. *See* Centers for Disease Control and
  Prevention
Center for Credentialing and Education, 22
Centers for Disease Control and
  Prevention (CDC), 120
Championing, 39–40
Change. *See* Behavior change
Change-resistance talk, 80, 118
Change talk, 80, 88–89, 118, 149
  amplified reflections and, 84
  empathy and, 81
  open-ended questions and, 82
  shifted-focus reflections and, 85
Character strengths. *See* Being skills;
  Signature strengths
Chartier, Emile, 151
Chronic contemplation, 15
Chronic diseases, 3, 7, 174
Chronic stress, 8, 63
Citizenship, 52
Client assessments. *See* Assessments
Clients
  confidence and, 118, 151
  emotional fitness of, 118
  energy levels of, 118, 123
  health of, 118, 123
  learning styles of, 5, 122
  life satisfaction of, 64, 118, 124
  mental fitness of, 118
  motivations for seeking coaching, 10
  nutrition and, 118, 123
  personality preferences of, 116
  physical activity and exercise of, 118, 123
  priorities of, 118
  professional conduct with, 23–24
  readiness for change of, 118–119
  stress and, 123

  support for, during change, 102–104
  trust and rapport with, 31
  weight management of, 118, 123
Closed-ended questions, 6, 35
Coaches. *See also* Coach training
  business, 1
  empathy for, 60–62
  life, 1, 2, 44
  need for, 2–5
  role of, 127
  self-care for, 19
Coaching
  assessments for, 115–118
  change, skills for, 101t, 102t
  clients' motivations for seeking, 10
  coach approach integration to, 9
  defined, 1–2
  executive, 1, 2
  expert approach and, 4, 5–7, 6t
  generative moments and, 143–145
  positivity and, 64–65
  process of, 8–9
  research on, 7
  therapy, distinguishing from, 20
Coaching agreement, 126–129, 128t
  coaching principles, 127–128
  "right" way and, 127
  role of coach, 127
  startup session, 128–129
  trust and, 127
Coaching presence
  being skills and, 44–49, 44f
  conveying, 49
  defining, 43–44
  signature strengths and, 49–53
Coaching program, 126
  feedback survey for, 168–171
  guidelines for
    close, 167
    ongoing coaching program, 166–167
    program startup, 165–166
    prospect stage, 165
  refresh or close of, 164
Coaching psychology
  defined, 11
  mechanisms in action
    confidence, 15
    growth-promoting relationships, 12–14
    process of change, 15–16
    self-motivation, 14–15
  self-determination and, 11–12
Coaching relationship, 74
Coaching relationship skills, 28f
  core skills of
    mindful listening and, 34–35
    open-ended inquiry and, 35–37
    perceptive reflections and, 37–38
  mindfulness and, 32–34
  relationship and, 27–29
  relationship-building tools and, 38–40
  trust and rapport and, 29–32
Coaching science. *See* Coaching psychology
Coaching sessions
  challenges and, 162–164

  close of, 162, 163t
  generative moments and, 162, 162t
  goal or experiment review and,
    158–161, 159t, 161t
  introduction to, 155–156
  opening of, 156–157, 157t
  preparing for, 156, 156t
  program refresh or close and, 164
*Coaching the Multiplicity of Mind:*
  *A Strengths-Based Approach*, 174
*Coaching World*, 174
Coach training
  becoming a coach
    learning, 17–18
    modeling and, 19–20
    practicing, 18
    professional development plan and,
      18–19
    self-care and, 19
  coaching and therapy, distinguishing,
    20
  liability and, 21–22
  other professionals, distinguishing
    from, 20–21
  scope of practice and, 21–22
CoachVille, 39, 47, 89
Coates, V., 155
Code of Ethics
  confidentiality and privacy, 24
  conflicts of interest, 23
  pledge of ethics, 24
  professional conduct at large, 22–23
  professional conduct with clients,
    23–24
Cognitive listening, 34
Cole, S., 3
Collaboration, 114–115
  design thinking and, 126
Compassion
  generative moments and, 143
  negative emotions and, 55–56
  nonviolent communication and, 58–62,
    62f
  self-compassion and, 57–58
  Self-Compassion Scale, 116
  self-esteem and, 56–57
Competence, 175–176
*The Complete Guide to Coaching at Work*
  (Zeus and Skiffington), 28
Conditioning, operant, 103–104
Confidence, 118, 151
  coaching psychology and, 15
  human thriving and, 175–176
  Mount Lasting Change Model and,
    108
  self-determination and, 15
Confidence ruler, 86, 87f
Confidentiality, 24, 32
Conflicts of interest, 23
Constructionist principle, 66
Consulting, 20–21
Contemplation stage, of change, 96–97
Controlled motivation, 78
Cooperrider, David, 65

Core Coaching Competencies, 100
Core values, 69
Corneae, Guy, 49
Courage
    as being skill, 48–49
    as signature strength, 51
Creativity, 16, 50
    human thriving and, 176
Crocker, B., 155
Csikszentmihalyi, Mihaly
    creativity and, 176
    flow and, 89, 152, 176
    self-efficacy and, 87, 91
Curiosity, 50, 123
    human thriving and, 176

**D**

Danner, D. D., 63
d'Ansembourg, Thomas, 49
Deci, Edward, 11, 14–15, 78, 79, 174–175
Decisional balance, 104–106, 116, 118
    change and, 82–83
    generative moments and, 149
Define phase, of AI, 68
De Haan, E., 28
Dementia, 176
Depression, 120
Design phase, of AI, 70–71
Design thinking, 132–135
    brainstorming and, 135–137
    coaching agreement and, 126–129,
        128t
    coaching program for, 126
    feedback on sessions and, 139
    intermediate behavioral goals and, 134
    nature of, 125–126
    outcomes progress, tracking and
        measuring of, 139
    planning and, 125
    visions and, 129–132, 131t, 132f
    weekly experiments and, 134–135, 135t
Destiny phase, of AI, 71
Deutschman, A., 79
Diabetes, 3, 7
Diagnostic and Statistical Manual of
    Mental Disorders, 5th edition (DSM-5),
    20, 50
DiClemente, Carlo, 100
Dill, D., 155
DISC (dominance, influence, steadiness,
    and compliance), 116, 122
Discovery phase, of AI, 68–70
Discrepancy, 114
    generative moments and, 149
    MI and, 82–84, 83f
Diseases
    Alzheimer, 86, 175, 176
    chronic, 3, 7, 174
    heart, 3, 7, 78
Distance live coaching, 9
Distress, 88
Dominance, influence, steadiness, and
    compliance. See DISC

Dotlich, David, 28
Double-sided reflections, 84
Dream phase, of AI, 70
DSM-5. See Diagnostic and Statistical
    Manual of Mental Disorders, 5th edition
Duvall, M., 152

**E**

Eating disorders, 120
Edington, Dee, 118
Edison, Thomas Alva, 155
Education, 21
EI. See Emotional intelligence
8 Colors of Fitness (Brue), 116
Emotional fitness, 118
Emotional indicators, for generative
    moments, 142, 142t
Emotional intelligence (EI), 113, 127, 152
Emotions
    high-road reactions, 56
    low-road reactions, 56
    mindfulness and, 33
    negative, 3, 45, 55–56, 64
    positive, 3, 15, 56
Empathy
    assessments and, 115
    as being skill, 45–46
    change talk and, 81
    for coach, 60–62
    defining, 58–59
    design thinking and, 126
    generative moments and, 143–144
    MI and, 81
    NVC and, 58–60
    physician, 55
    trust and rapport and, 29–30
Empathy reflections, 82
Energy levels, of clients, 118, 123
Environment, 73
    generative moments and, 148–149
    SCT and, 87
Envision brainset, 16
Ethics. See Code of Ethics
Eustress, 88
Evocative inquiry, 144
Excellence, appreciation of, 52–53
Executive coaching, 1, 2
Executive function, 176
Exercise, 118
Experiences
    best, 68–69
    mastery, 90–91
    new experience seeking, 176
    vicarious, 89–90
Experimentalism, 126
Expert approach, 4, 5–7, 6t
Expert hat, 114–115
External motivation, 14, 78

**F**

Fairness, 52
Faux feelings, 59

Feedback survey, for coaching program,
    168–171
Feelings. See also Emotions
    faux, 59
    needs-related, 61t
    personal, 60
First law of motion, 66
Fitness, mental and emotional, 118
Fitness industry, 4
5-D cycle of AI, 67–71, 67f
    define, 68
    design, 70–71
    destiny, 71
    discover, 68–70
    dream, 70
Five Facet Mindfulness Scale, 116
Flaste, R., 175
Flow, 77, 89, 127, 176
    relational, 16, 151–152
    studies, 152
    zone, 40, 88
Ford, Henry, 77, 175
Forgiveness, 52
Frankl, Viktor, 175
Fredrickson, Barbara, 116, 175
    meaning and purpose and, 3
    positive emotions and, 15, 56, 64
Friesen, W. V., 63
"From Surviving to Thriving" (article), 174
Future-oriented autonomous motivation, 14

**G**

Galantino, M., 156
Gallwey, Tim, 28, 43
Generative conditions, 69
Generative moments, 162, 162t
    coaching skills and
        brainstorming, 144–145
        compassion, 143
        empathy, 143–144
        evocative inquiry, 144
        mindful listening and, 144
        open-ended inquiry and, 144
        perceptive reflections, 144
        silence, 144
        unfailing affirmation and, 145
    defining, 141–142
    emotional indicators for, 142, 142t
    facilitating
        asking permission to explore topic
            and, 146–147
        brainstorming and, 149–151
        confidence in client, 151
        decisional balance and, 149
        discrepancy and, 149
        environments and, 148–149
        identifying topics and, 145–146
        strengths or values and, 147–148
    occurrences of, 142–143
    relational flow in, 151–152
Goals and goal setting. See Behavioral goals
Goethe, 141
Goleman, Daniel, 56, 152

Gordon, Thomas, 7
Grant, Anthony, 11
Gratitude, 53
Growth-promoting relationships, 12–14, 28, 44
Gruber, J., 64

**H**
Hall, L. M., 152
Harvard Health Publications, 174
Harvard Medical School, 47
Health and fitness industry, 4
Healthcare costs, 3–4
Health Insurance Portability and Accountability Act (HIPAA), 32, 121, 127
Health risk assessments (HRAs), 114
Heart disease, 3, 7, 78
Hettler, Bill, 115
High-road reactions, 56
Hill, M., 155
HIPAA. *See* Health Insurance Portability and Accountability Act
Hope, 53
HRAs. *See* Health risk assessments
Humanity, 51–52
Human thriving
    autonomy and, 174–175
    body regulation and, 174
    confidence and competence and, 175–176
    creativity and, 176
    curiosity and new experience seeking and, 176
    executive function and, 176
    meaning and purpose and, 175
    relationships and, 175
    standard setting and, 176–177
Humility, 30, 52
Humor, 39, 53
Humphrey, Holley, 81
Hunt, Diana Scharf, 125

**I**
"I am" stage, of change, 98–99
"I can't" stage, of change, 94–96
ICF. *See* International Coach Federation
Identity-oriented autonomous motivation, 14
"I may" stage, of change, 96–97
*The Inner Game of Work* (Gallwey), 28
Institute of Coaching, McLean Hospital, 7
Integrity, 51
Intelligence
    body, 45, 174
    emotional, 113, 127, 152
    social, 51–52
International Coach Federation (ICF), 8, 18, 20, 27–28, 100, 174. *See also* Code of Ethics
    coaching presence and, 43
    coaching sessions and, 155
    creating awareness and, 114

learning styles and, 122
    planning and, 125
    training and, 17
Interviewing. *See* Motivational interviewing
*The Introduction to NVC* (Kendrick), 60
Intuition, 120–121
"I still am" stage, of change, 99–100
"I will" stage, of change, 97–98
"I won't" stage, of change, 94–96

**J**
Judge, D., 155
Jung, Carl, 65
Justice, 52

**K**
Kabat-Zinn, Jon, 33, 35
Kashdan, Todd, 176
Kauffman, Carol, 47
Kawarau Bridge, 89
Kaye, M., 155
Kelm, Jacqueline Bascobert, 66
Kendrick, Greg, 60
Kindness, 51
Knowledge, 50–51

**L**
Lambert, M., 28
Lapses, in behavioral change, 99
Lasting change, 109
Latham, G. P., 133, 135
Laughter clubs, 48
Leadership, 52
Learning
    coach training and, 17–18
    love of, 51
    reflective, 100
    styles of, 5, 122
Leonard, Thomas, 44
Lerner, Harriet, 55
Liability, 21–22
Life coaches, 1, 2, 44
Life satisfaction, 64, 118, 124
Life skills, 4
Lifestyle medicine, 3
Lisowski, C., 155
Listening
    affective, 34
    cognitive, 34
    mindful, 34–35, 144
    perceptive reflections and, 37–38
    silence and, 39
Locke, E. A., 133, 135
Love, 51, 72–73
*Love 2.0: How Our Supreme Emotion Affects Everything We Feel, Think, Do, and Become* (Fredrickson), 175
Love of learning, 51
Low goals, 135
Low-road reactions, 56

**M**
MAAS. *See* Mindful Attention Awareness Scale
Maintenance stage, of change, 99–100
*Man's Search for Meaning* (Frankl), 175
Mastery experiences, 90–91
Mauss, I., 64
McGloin, H., 155
McLean Hospital, 7
Meaning, 3
    human thriving and, 175
    MI and, 85–86
Measurable goals, 133
Mental fitness, 118
Mentoring, 21
Mercy, 52
MI. *See* Motivational interviewing
Michelangelo, 1, 13
Miller, W., 80
Mindful Attention Awareness Scale (MAAS), 116
Mindful listening, 34–35
    generative moments and, 144
Mindfulness, 3, 13
    as being skill, 44–45, 45f
    coaching relationships and, 32–34
    Five Facet Mindfulness Scale, 116
Mindset, change of, 93
Modeling, 19–20
Modesty, 52
Motion, first law of, 66
Motivation
    autonomous, 14, 78–80, 175
    controlled, 78
    external, 14, 78
    self-efficacy and, 77, 86–91
        mastery experiences and, 90–91
        physiological or affective states, 88
        SCT and, 87–88
        verbal persuasion and, 88–89
        vicarious experiences and, 89–90
    self-motivation, 14–15
    visions and, 129–132
    well-being assessments and, 118–119, 121
Motivational interviewing (MI), 77, 127, 133
    engaging
        open-ended inquiry and, 82
        perceptive reflections and, 82
        resistance and, 80–82
    evoking
        meaning and, 85–86
        rulers and, 86, 87f
    focusing, 82–85
        discrepancy and, 82–84, 83f
        perceptive reflections and, 84–85
    generative moments and, 147
    planning, 86, 90–91
Mount Lasting Change Model, 93, 106–109, 107f, 114
    action level of, 109
    best self and, 109
    preparation level of, 108–109

results level of, 109
vision level of, 106–108
Murray, W. H., 151
Mutual care, 72
Myers Briggs Type Indicator, 116, 122

**N**
Nanus, Burt, 67
National Commission for Health
  Education Credentialing, 20
National Consortium for Credentialing
  Health & Wellness Coaches, 7
Needs, universal, 60
Needs-related feelings, 61t
Neff, Kristin, 56, 57, 116
Negative emotions, 3, 45, 55–56, 64
Nelson, H., 125
Neuroplasticity, 13–14
New experience seeking, 176
Newton, 66
No-fault zone, 145
Nonviolent communication (NVC),
  58–62, 62f, 77, 127
Norcross, J., 15, 28
Nutrition, 118, 123
NVC. *See* Nonviolent communication

**O**
Obesity, 3, 7
Open awareness, 45
Open-ended questions, 6, 35–37
  generative moments and, 144
  MI and, 82
Open-mindedness, 50–51
Operant conditioning, 103–104
Optimism, 126
Ornish, Dean, 79
Outcomes, tracking and measuring
  progress of, 139
Over-delivering, 30–31

**P**
Perceptive reflections, 37–38
  generative moments and, 144
  MI and, 82, 84–85
Performance goals, 16
PERMA model of well-being, 64
Perry, Jay, 19
Persistence, 51
Personal factors, in SCT, 87
Personal feelings, 60
Personality preferences, 116
Personal training, 21
Perspective, 51
Persuasion, verbal, 88–89
Peterson, C., 50, 63, 148
Phillips, E., 155
Phone conference coaching, 8
Physical activity, 118, 123
Physician empathy, 55
Physiological states, 88

Pity, 58–59
Playfulness
  as being skill, 48
  as relationship-building tool, 39
Poetic principle, 67
Point A to point B, 2, 3f, 155
Pojednic, R., 155
Polak, R., 5, 155
Porges, Stephen W., 174
Positive emotions, 3, 15, 56
Positive frame, 73–74
Positive principle, 66
Positive psychology, 63–64, 127, 173
  AI and
    coaching relationship and, 74
    5-D cycle of, 67–71, 67f
    five principles of, 65–67, 65f
    value of, 71–72
  coaching and, 64–65
  problem solving and, 72–74
Positive reframing, 38–39
Positive regard, 46
  unconditional, 29
*Positivity* (Fredrickson), 64
Positivity Ratio, 116
Precontemplation stage, of change, 94–96
Prediabetes, 3
Preparation level, of Mount Lasting
  Change Model
    commitment, 108
    confidence, 108
    plan, 108–109
    support, 108
Preparation stage, of change, 97–98
Privacy, 24
Problem solving, 72–74, 109
Prochaska, James, 93, 94, 100
Professional conduct
  with clients, 23–24
  at large, 22–23
Professional development plan, 18–19
Progress reports, 16
Prolepsis, 66
Prudence, 52
Psychology. *See* Coaching psychology;
  Positive psychology
Psychotherapy, 28
Purpose, 3, 85–86, 175

**Q**
Quality of Life Inventory, 116
Questions. *See also* Appreciative inquiry
  closed-ended, 6, 35
  open-ended, 6, 35–37, 82, 144
Quickie Well-Being Assessment, 116, 117f

**R**
Rapport
  authenticity and, 32
  client and, 31
  coaching sessions and, 156
  confidentiality and, 32

empathy and, 29–30
  role models and, 30
  slowing down and, 30
  unconditional positive regard and, 29
  under-promising and over-delivering
    and, 30–31
  well-being assessments and, 121
Readiness ruler, 86, 87f
Readiness to change, 118–119
  assessment, 104, 105t, 152
Realistic goals, 133
Reappraisal, 56
Red flags, 114
Referrals, 114, 120
Reflections
  amplified, 84
  double-sided, 84
  empathy, 82
  perceptive, 37–38, 82, 84–85, 114
  shifted-focus, 85
  simple, 84
Reflective learning, 100
Reflective practitioner, 152
Reframing, positive, 38–39
Relapse prevention, 109
Relatedness, 29
Relational competence, 152
Relational flow, 16, 151–152
Relationship-building tools
  championing and, 39–40
  humor and, 39
  input and suggestions and, 40
  playfulness and, 39
  positive reframing and, 38–39
  silence and, 39
Relationships, 175. *See also* Coaching
  relationship skills
Relaxation techniques, 33
Reminder techniques, 33
Resilience, 64
Resistance, in MI, 80–82
Responsibility, 107
Results level, of Mount Lasting Change
  Model
    lasting change, 109
    relapse prevention, 109
Rewards, 109
Rhode, Robert, 149
Righting reflex, 81
Roberts, P., 155
Rogers, Carl, 29, 60
Role models, 19, 30
Rollnick, S., 80
Rosenberg, Marshall, 58, 60, 81
Roy, B., 155
Rulers, 86, 87f
Rumi, 85
Rush Alzheimer's Disease Center, 175
Ryan, Richard, 11, 14–15, 79, 116, 174–175

**S**
Schwartz, J., 155
Science, 91

Scope of practice, 21–22
SCT. *See* Social cognitive theory
Self-awareness, 107
Self-care, for coach, 19
Self-change, 94
Self-compassion, 57–58
Self-Compassion Scale, 116
Self-concept, 6
Self-criticism, 55
Self-determination, 8, 58, 127, 139, 173, 175
    coaching psychology and, 11–12
    coaching relationship and, 29
    confidence and, 15
    generative moments and, 149
Self-directed neuroplasticity, 13
Self-efficacy, 5, 12, 15, 175
    change and, 103
    motivation and, 77, 86–91
        mastery experiences and, 90–91
        physiological or affective states, 88
        SCT and, 87–88
        verbal persuasion and, 88–89
        vicarious experiences and, 89–90
        well-being assessments and, 118–119
Self-esteem, 56–57
Self-image, 102
Self-kindness, 57
Self-motivation, 14–15
Self-regulation, 52
    generative moments and, 148–149
Self-sabotage, 73
Seligman, M. E. P., 50, 63, 64, 148, 173
Sforzo, G., 155
Sherman, R., 155
Shifted-focus reflections, 85
Signature strengths, 49–53
    courage and, 51
    humanity and, 51–52
    justice, 52
    temperance, 52
    transcendence, 52–53
    wisdom and knowledge, 50–51
Signature Strengths Questionnaire, 45, 50, 116
Silberman, J., 45
Silence, 49
    generative moments and, 144
    listening and, 39
Silsbee, Doug, 28
Simple reflections, 84
Simultaneity principle, 66
Six dimensions of wellness model, 115, 115f
Skiffington, Suzanne, 28
SMART goals, 16, 71, 133
Smoking cessation study, 79–80
Snowdon, D. A., 63
Social cognitive theory (SCT), 77, 87–88
*Social Foundations of Thought and Action: A Social Cognitive Theory* (Bandura), 87
Social intelligence, 51–52
Social norms, 102

Spirituality, 53
Standard setting, 176–177
Stevens, Nicola, 39
Stolterman, E., 125
Storytelling, 36
Strengths, 107
    generative moments and, 147–148
    signature, 49–53
StrengthsFinder, 50
Stress, 88, 123
    burnout and, 19
    chronic, 8, 63
    management interventions for, 3
Strokes, 3
Strozzi Heckler, Richard, 146
Substance abuse, 120
Success, acknowledgment of, 74
Sympathy, 58–59

**T**
Talbert, M., 155
Tamir, M., 64
Temperance, 52
Therapy, 21
    coaching, distinguishing from, 20
    psychotherapy, 28
Three-month behavioral goals, 134, 134t
    check-in for, 159–161, 161t
Three wishes, 69–70
Thriving. *See* Human thriving
Thurman, Howard, 173
Timmons, F., 155
Training, 21. *See also* Coach training
Transcendence, 52–53
Transtheoretical Model of Change (TTM), 15, 90, 93–94, 100, 118, 133
Trial and correction, 74
Trust
    authenticity and, 32
    client and, 31
    coaching agreement and, 127
    coaching sessions and, 156
    confidentiality and, 32
    empathy and, 29–30
    role models and, 30
    slowing down and, 30
    unconditional positive regard and, 29
    under-promising and over-delivering and, 30–31
    well-being assessments and, 121
Tschannen-Moran, Megan, 29
TTM. *See* Transtheoretical Model of Change

**U**
Unconditional positive regard, 29
Under-promising, 30–31
Unfailing affirmation, 145
Universal needs, 60
University of Rochester, 11
University of Sydney, 11

U.S. Department of Health and Human Services, 32
U.S. National Wellness Institute, 115

**V**
Values, 108
    of AI, 71–72
    of assessments, 113–115
    core, 69
    generative moments and, 147–148
Values-in-Action (VIA), 45, 50, 116
Verbal persuasion, 88–89
VIA. *See* Values-in-Action
Vicarious experiences, 89–90
Video conference coaching, 8–9
"Viktor Frankl's Meaning Seeking Model and Positive Psychology" (Wong), 175
Virtues, 50
Vision level, of Mount Lasting Change Model, 106–108
    benefits and information, 108
    challenges and strategies, 108
    self-awareness and responsibility, 107
    strengths, 107
    values, 108
Visions, in design thinking
    drawing and, 132f
    examples of, 132
    motivation and, 129–132
    protocol for designing, 131t
    visualization tool for, 131t
Vitality, 51

**W**
Walker, David, 3
Warmth, 46
Weatherhead School of Management, 65
Weekly experiments, 134–135, 135t
Weight loss counseling, 5–6
Weight management, 118, 123
Well-being assessments
    AI and, 121–122
    discussing components of, 122–124
    exploring results of, 119–120
    intuition and, 120–121
    learning styles and, 122
    motivation and, 118–119, 121
    trust and rapport and, 121
Wheatley, Margaret, 67
Wheel of life, 113, 116, 116f
Willingness ruler, 86, 87f
Wisdom, 50–51
Wolever, R., 7
Wong, Paul, 85, 175
Working alliance, 28

**Z**
Zander, Benjamin, 48, 66
Zander, Rosamund Stone, 48, 66
Zest, 47–48
Zeus, Perry, 28